NOURISH

The beginner's guide to
eating healthy and staying fit

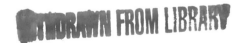

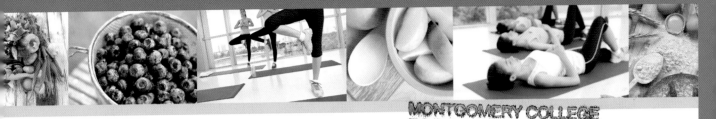

NOURISH

The beginner's guide to
eating healthy and staying fit

Front Table Books • An imprint of Cedar Fort, Inc. • Springville, Utah

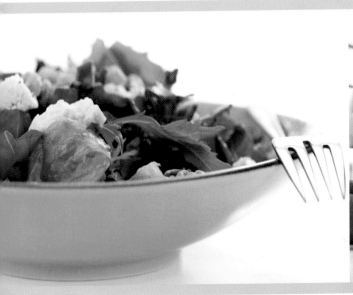

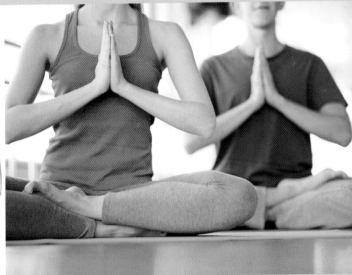

CHRISTI SILBAUGH

ISBN 13: 978-1-4621-1552-5

Published by Front Table Books, an imprint of Cedar Fort, Inc.
2373 W. 700 S., Springville, UT 84663
Distributed by Cedar Fort, Inc., www.cedarfort.com

LIBRARY OF CONGRESS CATALOGING-IN-PUBLICATION DATA

Silbaugh, Christi.
Nourish / Christi Silbaugh.
      pages cm
Includes index.
ISBN 978-1-4621-1552-5 (acid-free paper)
1. Nutrition. 2. Reducing diets. 3. Yoga. I. Title.

RA784.S538 2015
641.5'635--dc23

2014043841

Cover design by Lauren Error
Cover design © 2015 Lyle Mortimer
Edited by Justin Greer

Printed in China

10 9 8 7 6 5 4 3 2 1

Printed on acid-free paper

THIS BOOK IS DEDICATED TO ALL THOSE WHO ARE READY TO COMMIT TO HAVING A HAPPY, HEALTHY LIFE.

FOREWORD: THE JOY OF MOVEMENT

It doesn't need to be a difficult act. It's simply moving your body. You don't need to get up and down; what I encourage is the sheer act of bringing the joy of movement to your body.

As a yoga instructor, I can't tell you the numerous times I hear people dismiss the idea of yoga because they say that they are not flexible enough or they express fear that they will look foolish amongst others. The truth is, we all have to start somewhere. Movement—whether it takes place on a yoga mat, at your desk at work, or down on the ground—can have profound affects on both your external body as well as your internal. Accompanied with breath, movement not only circulates the blood, but it circulates and stirs up any unnecessary energies harboring inside. It rids the body of toxins, rinsing out both the unhealthy foods and drinks we put in our body as well as the negative biases of the mind. It can bring balance when we feel rocked; it can help alter and shift perspectives; it goes beyond just moving the body; it's about connecting to ourselves and being our own solution for this hectic and hurried life.

What are you doing to take care and nourish the most important person of your life both internally and externally? What kinds of thoughts and foods are you digesting? What simple changes can you bring to your life towards creating positive change? How are you practicing self-love?

Take one step. Today, create space in your schedule to move. Bring balance, breath, and growth into your heart, into your mind, and into your body through the nourishing act of movement. Are you ready and willing?

Be on your own side and cultivate positive changes in your life.

Love flows,
Heather Foat

CONTENTS

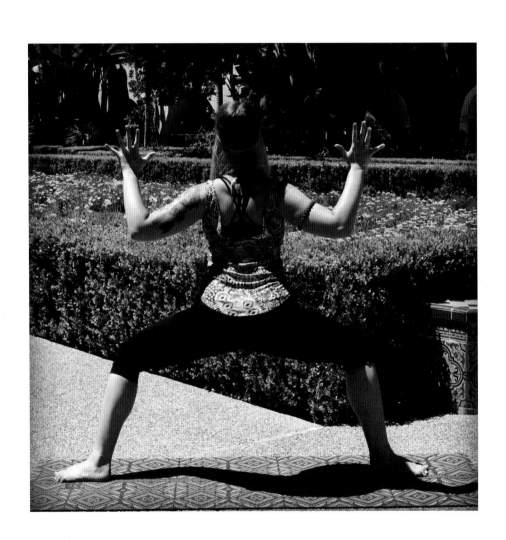

INTRODUCTION

In life, you learn lessons along the way. When you are in elementary, middle, and high school, your parents, teachers, and coaches help you learn how to eat right, move your body, and stay committed. Then, some of you go right to work straight from high school. Others go to college. The very few continue to play sports in college, and that is why gaining 15 pounds during your freshman year is so common. No one tells you to move anymore. No one balances your meals. You are on your own in the world with very little education on real food. You are pressed for time in a world packed with preservatives, chemicals, and processed foods.

After a few years you realize the damage, and then the cycle starts and continues with radical diets and up-and-down failures. We see numerous commercials for prepackaged foods that are low-fat and low-calorie. We are told time and time again that it is *calories in* and *calories out* that count. The truth is, this is false. While calories do matter, it is time we count chemicals and quality of calories, not just calories. Somewhere along the way things got skewed. We blindly started eating non-food contaminates in place of whole foods. We got busy and needed to grab and go. From generation to generation the bad habits have been handed down. It is almost to the point that people don't even recognize real food anymore.

I am just as guilty as anyone when it comes to following the traditions and just eating what I see. I have been on the yo-yo diet insanity cycle. I have devoured my share of processed food and sugar-packed treats. That all changed for me though. I unfortunately got my education on this matter the hard way. I am a cancer survivor. I am happy today to tell you I am cancer free and stronger than ever, thanks to good doctors that cared enough to educate me on proper diet and exercise. I am writing this book to help prevent others from having to deal with sickness. I believe the answer is whole foods and movement in your body.

When I started my recovery, I felt at my all-time low. I was overweight from being too sick to have movement in my body, and the tumor in my uterus had caused my belly to look pregnant. I felt like I had no muscle mass. My kind doctor saw my frustration. I wanted to start working out, but had little strength and no self confidence. I was told to start yoga. It is reconstructive and a healing exercise. So I did. I found a local, small-community yoga studio called Pura Vida Yoga in San Diego. I first went three times per week, and worked my way up to six days a week. Within six months I had lost all of my cancer weight and felt stronger than ever. By eating whole foods and doing yoga I had gained my life back.

I started to reflect back on things and realized I had passed on to my kids the same bad habits passed on to me. I always cooked at home, so they had not been faced with the bad out-to-eat choices before leaving the nest. At the start of writing this book, my kids were 20 and 21, and they were making the same bad food choices all the other kids their age were. They thought Jamba Juice was a healthy choice. Something had to be done. I started talking to them and their friends. I gathered information from my doctor, nutrition and the young adults themselves.

My goal with this book is to show you how you can eat healthy and exercise on a budget, to make sure you realize that you cannot out-exercise a bad diet, and to introduce you to real whole foods that taste amazing and are easy to make.

I have gathered my favorite healthy whole food recipes, yoga poses, inspirational quotes, and lots of pictures to help you on your journey. So let's get started!

4 STEPS TO A HEALTHIER YOU

STEP 1: CLEAN OUT THE FRIDGE AND PANTRY!

I know you are probably not happy about getting rid of food you spent your hard-earned money on. Nevertheless, it has to be done. Chances are, if you bought this book, you are looking for a change. The definition of insanity is doing the same thing over and over and expecting a different result. So I need you to trust me. If you bought your food at a big supermarket chain, it is most likely that your fridge and pantry are full of non-food items that you have been eating your whole life.

Today, more than three-quarters of supermarket shelves are stocked with packaged and processed foods. These boxed, canned, and frozen concoctions are full of more than 3,000 food chemicals purposely added to our food supply. You probably already know this, but the best foods to stay healthy are unprocessed natural foods. That's because man-made chemicals

acidify your body pH. Would you eat your favorite breakfast cereal if you knew that it contained butylated hydroxytoluene (BHT), a product also used in jet fuel and embalming fluid? Can you imagine grilling your low-fat veggie burger if you found out that its main ingredient is monosodium glutamate (MSG)?

Read the label. Please be careful, because foods that are considered "healthy" and labeled as "natural" contain many harmful chemicals and non-food ingredients (like wood shavings) used as food preservatives and flavor enhancers—and these chemicals are often disguised under unrecognizable names.

Because I know you can't possibly remember 3,000 chemicals, I am going to give you what I consider the seven worst offenders and why.

BHT (butylated hydroxytoluene): This is an additive used to prevent oxidation in a wide variety of foods and cosmetics. It is listed by the National Toxicology Program (NTP) in 2005 as "reasonably anticipated to be a human carcinogen" on the basis of experimental findings in animals. It is also used in jet fuels, rubber petroleum products, transformer oil, and embalming fluid. As if this were not enough, the Material Safety Data Sheet (MSDS) warns that BHT should not be allowed to enter the environment, can cause liver damage, and is harmful to aquatic organisms. (You can find out more information on the NTP website, ntp.niehs.nih.gov, and you can see the MSDS by searching for BHT at www.msdsonline.com/msds-search.)

High Fructose Corn Syrup (HFCS): Studies have shown that the reactive carbonyl molecules can cause tissue damage that may lead to obesity, diabetes, and heart disease. To make matters worse, studies have recently revealed that nearly half of tested samples of HFCS contained mercury. (Information is available from Food Politics at www.foodpolitics.com/wp-content/uploads/HFCS_Rats_10.pdf and from a Princeton study at http://www.princeton.edu/main/news/archive/S26/91/22K07/.)

Yellow #5: Almost all colorants approved for use in food are derived from coal tar and may contain up to 10 ppm of lead and arsenic. Coal tar colors have been proven to potentially cause cancer. (Information can be found in a www.saveourbones.com article by Vivian Goldschmidt, MA.)

Soybean oil: More than half of all soybean crops grown in the US are genetically modified (GMO). There is a growing concern and mounting scientific evidence that genetic engineering of food plant seeds may have an unexpected and negative impact on human health. On a side note, this is also why you should be buying organic food. (To find out more, read the article by Le Rockwell found at www.lewrockwell.com/2013/01/joseph-mercola/soybean-oil-one-of-the-most-harmful-ingredients-in-processed-foods/.)

Propylene glycol alginate (E405): This food thickener, stabilizer, and emulsifier is derived from alginic acid esterified and combined with propylene glycol. Even though propylene glycol is allowed to be used as an additive in food, it is also used as an automotive antifreeze and airport runway deicer. Yum yum! Information can be found in the same www.saveourbones.com article by Vivian Goldschmidt, MA.)

Polysorbate 60: This is short for polyoxyethylene (20) sorbitan monostearate, an emulsifier made of corn, palm oil, and petroleum. This gooey mix can't spoil, so it often replaces dairy products in baked goods and other liquid products. If the box said "contains petroleum," would you eat it?

Textured soy protein concentrate, carrageenan, maltodextrin, disodium inosinate, disodium guanylate, and modified cornstarch: These are industry names for monosodium glutamate (MSG) (or they form MSG during processing). MSG and its related products have been linked to skin rashes, nausea, migraine headaches, heart irregularities, and even seizures.

I know that is probably overwhelming to read, and that is only seven of the bad ones. After being educated on this fact during my cancer struggle and being told no one should be eating these items, I knew something had to be done! I don't want to have to scare you straight, but they are now saying that by the year 2040 50% of America will have developed some form of cancer (see http://www.cnn.com/2014/02/04/health/who-world-cancer-report/ and (http://www.ourstolenfuture.org/NEWSCIENCE/human/cancer/cancerincidence.htm). It is time to take control of what we are putting in our bodies. Unfortunately, the food industry only cares about money and not health.

My solution is to buy organic food whenever you can. Find local farmers and buy direct from farmers' markets whenever you possibly can. This will ensure affordable, high-quality food, and you are supporting a farmer. Read labels on food you do buy in markets. Most importantly, find a healthy market that sells food you can trust. Here in California we have Sprouts, Jimbo's, and Whole Foods. Unfortunately, I can only give you guidelines on what stores are in my area; they change vastly depending on what area you live in. There are also a lot of mom and pop shops that are getting on board the organic train. Even Costco has started carrying more organic products. Take a few minutes and research where you can shop for your good produce.

I also want to include something here that won't make me very popular, but it needs to be said. You need to stop buying Starbucks or any other syrup-filled drinks. I think you may have to live in a cave if you have not read Food Babe's breakdown of a pumpkin spice latte (which has a bunch of the bad ingredients listed above in it, and no real pumpkin in the drink whatsoever). I know it is a trend, but if you fill your body with a Starbucks, you are filling it with toxic chemicals. I know it is hard, but your health is so worth it! There are numerous DIY recipes online, my blog included, that give you solutions for making healthy coffee drinks that taste the same at home. They are cheaper, too, so that is a plus!

STEP 2: STOP MAKING EXCUSES

I have a headache. I am sore. I have cramps. I am too tired. I can pretty much guarantee that if you say any one of those, it is most likely caused by the food you have put in your body. I cannot stress enough that it always, always, always begins with food. If you hear yourself giving an excuse, try your best to know that things sometimes get worse before they get better. Detoxing from chemicals in our food can be a painful

process. The body is designed to feel good and powerful, but if we feed the machine with garbage, the body will shut down. If you can start thinking of food as fuel for your machine, it will change everything. The first week is the hardest. Find some support from friends and family or your local yoga studio and buckle down.

Let me give you a scenario. You have just purchased your dream car, whatever that car may be. It has an amazing engine. You put everything into that car. Would you fill it with the cheapest gas if the manual said to put in premium? Probably not, and if you did, soon you would notice wear and tear on the engine. It won't run as smooth, you may get worse gas mileage, and eventually you will have to take it in for repair—at which time you will be told not to put that into this fine piece of machinery.

This analogy applies to your body and food, unless you think that a car deserves to be cared for more than your body. In my opinion, your body is so much more important. You must try your best to retrain your mind. I realize we have all been taught bad habits our whole life, but it is never to late to fix it and start again.

STEP 3: LEARN TO REPLACE YOUR CRAVINGS WITH GOOD, WHOLESOME FOOD

You can have your cake and eat it too, as you will find in my healthy treats section. You see, once upon a time we did not have overprocessed foods. People still ate back then, they just ate whole, God-given foods. We learned to work with them, break them down, and make scrumptious meals. I am going back to that time for you. When you have healthy items on hand to grab when you are feeling weak, it will greatly improve your success rate.

STEP 4: MOVE YOUR BODY

I cannot stress enough that everyone needs to be moving their bodies every single day. In this book I am focusing on yoga, mostly because yoga is how I got my life back after cancer and it is for everyone. You can be 90 years old in a wheelchair and still do some yoga. While this book does not focus on chair yoga, I assure you that it is out there. In fact there is bed yoga, chair yoga, floor yoga, paddle board yoga, aerial yoga, acro yoga . . . the list goes on and on.

As the lovely Heather Foat wrote in the foreword, it can be as simple as raising your hands above your head and taking in a deep breath to get started. I know getting started is the hardest part, but I promise you that if you can get to a yoga class, or just do a yoga practice in the privacy of your home, you will feel so much better. Try to promise yourself you will move your body every day. Even if it is just 15 minutes, move.

I don't want to presume I know your situation. I can only tell you mine, and the observations I have made by interviewing numerous people on the health and weight loss battle. It is important to me that you know I was 50 pounds overweight. I could not even do one full push-up when I started my yoga journey. I tried boot camp workouts, gym memberships, and willpower. I always had a little success to start, but I would end up sick and sore and I would quit. While I think any and all exercise is good when done properly, I am telling you this to let you know I know all the excuses.

I have used them.

Yoga is the place to start because it is healing. It gives you quiet time with yourself to reflect and meditate. Yoga is the first exercise I have done that I have fallen in love with. Even if I am sore, I know that going to yoga will help with the soreness.

As I stated before, yoga is for everyone. It can also be done anywhere. As we put together the poses for this book, we decided to focus on the outdoors in an effort to show you it can be done anywhere. You don't need expensive equipment or a gym membership. I would like to encourage you to get to a studio when you can. Yoga teachers can see your body and help you with alignment. You also will find great love and support at a community yoga studio. I have found the most supportive friends that I now call family. You want as much support as you can get on your journey, and a yoga studio is a great place for that.

There are a lot of free resources out there for people wanting to learn yoga. YouTube is riddled with how-to videos and yoga flows, as are other numerous media outlets like grokker.com. The internet is there: use it!

THE POSES

I have rounded up some beginner, intermediate, and advanced yoga poses to stimulate your curiosity and hopefully get you to start trying out some yoga movement. While in classes, the poses will usually come in a flow. This is a way for you to learn what the poses are and slowly gain confidence so you feel you can attend a class. Please note that there are advanced postures to keep you motivated. I do not expect you to drop into a headstand immediately. It is, however, important to me that you know that, at the time of writing this book, I have only been doing yoga for 10 months. I fell in love and practice every day, and you will see me in numerous pictures throughout the book to prove to you that anyone can do it with practice and determination. Once you master the easy poses, start trying a few arm balances, and eventually you will be ready to go upside down.

Please note that we did our best to present you with proper alignment directions and photos, but we are human and we don't claim to be perfect! I cannot agree more with the words of Pattabhi Jois: "Practice and all is coming." We are still practicing. Please take the time to read the instructions rather than just following the picture. In most cases, the picture is the full expression of the pose, but even if you are just in step one of the pose, you are still doing it. Take your time and practice and eventually you will be doing all of the yoga poses in this book and more.

Your yoga journey is all about you. You will first start out with it being an exercise and then you will slowly find out more and more about yourself. It is called a journey because it is never over. There is always more, and that is the best part!

THE YOGIS

I want to take a minute and introduce to you the yogis modeling in this book. They've worked hard to bring you some great shots of poses for you to work on, so I want to give you a little information on how you can continue your journey with them.

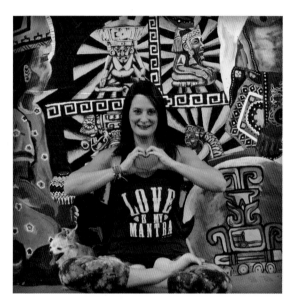

CHRISTI SILBAUGH

Yep, that's me! I am scattered through the book as a way to let you know anyone can do it. Before I started, I was 50 pounds overweight and had very little muscle mass. I am a 41-year-old mom. If I can do it, you can do it! If you want to meet me in person, I will be coming to your area soon doing NOURISH workshops. Follow me on Instagram @momwhatsfordinner to hear about the where and when and send me a shout-out. I can't wait to meet all of you!

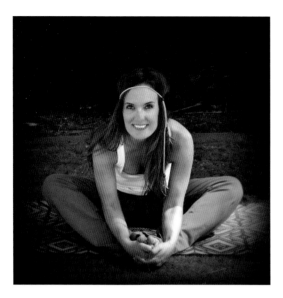

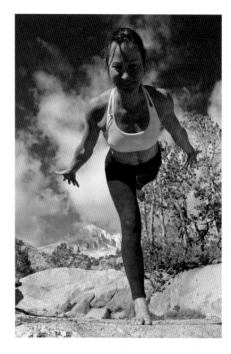

HEATHER FOAT

Heather Foat currently lives in her ideal life in San Diego, CA. She completed her 200-Hour Yoga Certification at Zuda Yoga in Sacramento, CA in 2010 and Prenatal/Postnatal 45-Hour Certification at Yoga Tree, San Francisco, CA in 2012. She actively pursues her love of yoga, music, and art. She instructs gentle flow yoga, prenatal and postnatal yoga, kids' yoga, and art and power vinyasa; she is passionate about creating spaces that are lighthearted and cultivate strength, the joy of movement, and self-love. Find out more information about her at www.Liv4yoga.com.

PAISLEY CLOSE

Paisley Close believes yoga is one of many paths to finding a deep sense of peace and contentment within. She's been teaching yoga since 2000 and makes it a priority to lead her students down this path of empowerment and freedom. Paisley pulls from rich real-life experiences to make the practice of yoga relatable both on and off the mat. She knows it's in the most challenging circumstances that we have the chance to cultivate strength, heal, and learn to love ourselves fully. Paisley is the author of two yoga books, *Healthy Shoulders: A Primer For Strengthening & Stretching* and *Headstand: From Basics to Balancing*. You can read Paisley's blog, purchase her books, and find out more about her at www.paisleyanne.com.

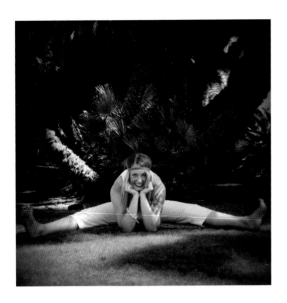

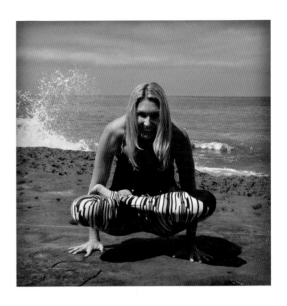

TAYLOR ANN SILBAUGH

Taylor Ann grew up in Oregon and moved to San Diego when she was in high school. She grew up playing basketball, singing, and playing guitar. Taylor is now in an internship for her incredible church, C3 San Diego, as a youth leader over all the beautiful junior high girls. She started yoga after her mother (the author of this book) was diagnosed with cancer and the doctors prescribed her yoga to help her get back on her feet. To be supportive, Taylor went to a yoga class with her where Heather Foat was teaching that morning. Taylor completely fell in love with the beauty, healing, and power that it gave her, being able to quiet her mind to actually listen to that still small voice that her pastors always spoke of but that she struggled so hard to hear. Yoga has inspired Taylor to become the leader God has called her to be for her girls, for her family, and most importantly for Jesus. You can follow her on Instagram @harmony527.

COURTNEY BERG

Growing up as a competitive athlete, Courtney has always made health and fitness a part of her life. Upon graduating from the University of Miami in 2004, she discovered yoga as a means to stay fit and strong. Her on-again, off-again relationship with yoga continued while trying to balance a demanding career in marketing and public relations in both agency and corporate settings. Over the years, yoga evolved from a more physical practice to one with a mental and spiritual connection for stress management, overall wellness, and inner peace. Having reached her "dream" job, Courtney realized she wanted more from life and to find a greater purpose to help others. In the summer of 2014, Courtney took time off while aiding a sick family member to reevaluate career and life aspirations, while reconnecting with self and losing 50 pounds. Yoga became her solace, and she received her RYT 200-Hour Certification, Interdisciplinary Vinyasa Flow, from Yoga One San Diego. She also became a Certified Worksite Wellness Specialist through the National Wellness Institute. A native of Arizona, Courtney currently resides in San Diego, CA, and is working to empower others to discover sustainable life-balance while looking beyond limitations and redefining a happier and healthier version of true self through yoga, creative marketing consulting, and corporate wellness. You can follow her journey at www.SixFootLiving.com and on Instagram @SixFootLiving.

ing spending a year abroad in Italy. In 2011, she was in a car accident that severely injured her back. After a couple of back procedures in 2014, she was finally able to return to her practice, and she received her RYT 200 from Yoga One that summer. She believes that yoga is an excellent way to connect with your true nature.

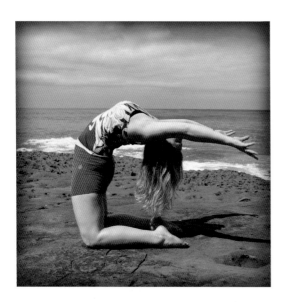

HALLEY HENSCEY

A San Francisco native, Halley Henscey started doing yoga with her parents when she was in preschool. She moved to San Diego to attend UCSD in 2004, where she studied linguistics and foreign languages, includ-

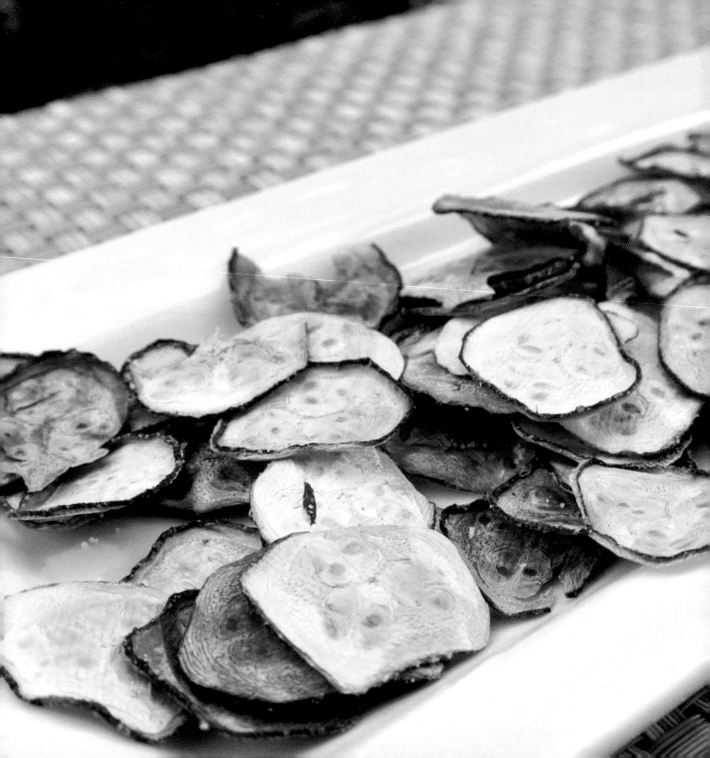

HEALTHY GRAB-AND-GO SNACKS

Being an active person on the go can really make it difficult to stick to healthy eating. Let's be honest: life is busy! With so many processed, gluten-free, prepackaged snack foods popping up on the shelves of our favorite markets, it seems like we are fighting a losing battle on the "eat whole foods" campaign. They are so easy to just grab and go that we all have given in to the convenience food temptation. They are not good for us, and we need to avoid them as much as possible.

The solution is to plan ahead. You do not need to be a fancy chef or have special strange ingredients in your pantry to make healthy, wholesome, on-the-go snacks that will nourish your body.

Let the Healthy Grab-and-Go Snacks section be your answer and have it take the temptation away. These recipes for healthy snacks, that you can make in bulk ahead of time with simple common ingredients, will give you energy and keep you satisfied—and some will even curb your sweet tooth!

Don't get discouraged when you have the urge to snack. Just keep a lot of healthy snacks available to you.

APPLE CHIPS

Serves 2

2 large Granny Smith apples
canola oil cooking spray
1 teaspoon cinnamon
1 teaspoon stevia

Preheat oven to 200 degrees F.

Thinly slice apples crosswise with a mandoline or sharp knife, as thin as you can. Arrange apple slices in a single layer baking sheet and spray with canola oil cooking spray.

Sprinkle cinnamon and stevia evenly over apple slices.

Bake in the top or bottom third of the oven until the apples are dry and crisp, about 2–2.5 hours.

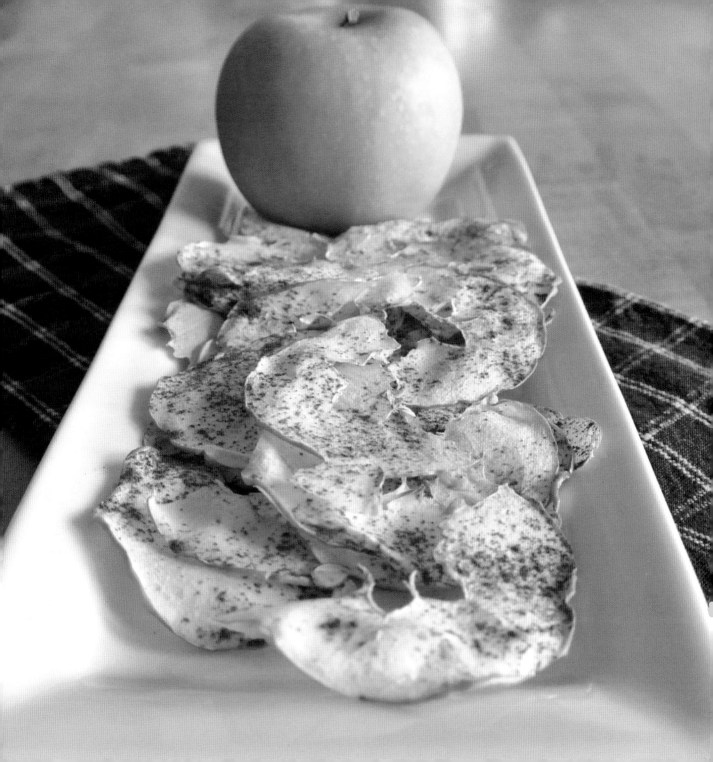

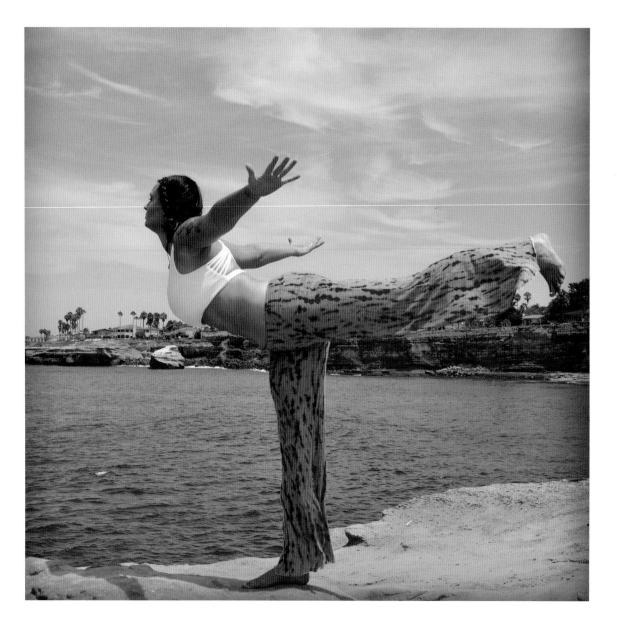

Top by Paramita Flow Designs – etsy.com/shop/paramitaflowdesigns
Pants by Liza and Jane Handmade – etsy.com/shop/lizajanehandmade

"Courage doesn't always roar. Sometimes courage is the quiet voice at the end of the day saying, 'I will try again tomorrow.'"
– MARY ANNE RADMACHER

AIRPLANE POSE

Begin in Mountain Pose (page 17).

Extend arms out to either side.

When you feel balanced, exhale and lean forward, lifting one leg straight behind you.

Hold this pose, then return your leg to the ground and your arms to your sides. Remember to always repeat on the other side.

Growing up I thought I disliked asparagus. Turns out I just don't like it overcooked. Raw is even better. Give it a try!

SHAVED ASPARAGUS SALAD

Serves 2

12 ounces asparagus, trimmed
2 tablespoons Bragg's amino acid
1 tablespoon fresh lemon juice
sea salt and freshly ground black pepper to taste
1 cup of your favorite lettuce

Shave asparagus into long thin strands using a vegetable peeler or mandoline. Soak the strands in a large bowl of ice water for one hour. Drain well and dry with paper towels.

To make the dressing, combine Bragg's amino acid, lemon juice, salt, and pepper to taste in a small bowl. Whisk until blended. Pour the dressing over the asparagus and toss well. Arrange over a bed of lettuce. Serve immediately.

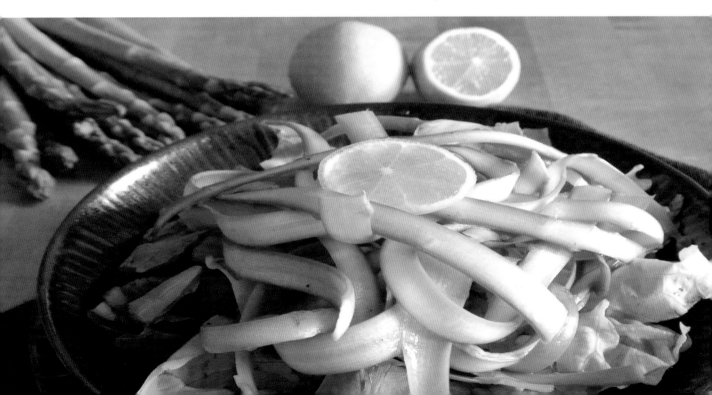

MOUNTAIN POSE

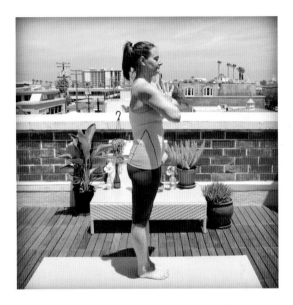

Come to stand with the big toes touching. The feet may be up to hips-distance apart if you need.

Lift up all your toes and let them fan out, then drop them down, creating a wide, solid base.

Let the feet and the calves root down into the floor.

Engage the quadriceps and draw them upward, causing your kneecaps to rise.

Rotate both thighs inward, creating a widening of the sit bones. Maintain the natural curves of your spine.

Outfit by Green Apple Activewear – greenappleactive.com
Mat by Manduka – manduka.com

Tone the belly, drawing it in slightly.

Widen the collar bones and make sure the shoulders are parallel to the pelvis.

The neck is long, the crown of the head rises toward the ceiling, and the shoulder blades slide down the back.

It may seem like you are just standing there, but bringing the body into proper alignment is hard work. The alignment for Mountain Pose leads into many of the standing and inverted poses, so this is considered the most important yoga pose to learn.

If you are a fan of traditional hummus, you are going to love this extra creamy avocado hummus filled with nutrients.

AVOCADO HUMMUS

Serves 4

2 avocados, peeled and chopped
1 (15-ounce) can chickpeas, drained and rinsed
¼ cup fresh lemon juice
2 tablespoons tahini
½ cup extra-virgin olive oil,
          plus more for drizzling
kosher salt
freshly ground pepper

In a food processor, add the avocados with the chickpeas, lemon juice, tahini, and olive oil, and purée until smooth; season with salt and pepper.

Transfer the dip to a bowl, drizzle with olive oil, and serve with veggies, bread, and chips.

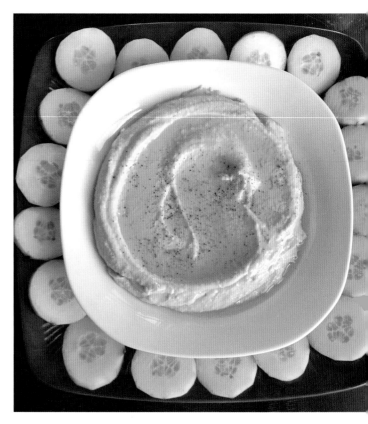

> "If you cannot do great things, do small things in a great way."
> **– NAPOLEON HILL**

STANDING SIDE BEND

Start in Mountain Pose (page 17). Inhale and raise your arms overhead, hands facing each other. Grab your left wrist with your right hand gently.

Exhale and bend your upper body to the right. Hold for several breaths. Inhale and bring the body back to the original position. Repeat on the other side.

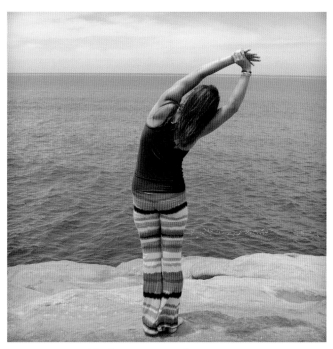

Top by Be Present – bepresent.com
Pants by Liza Jane Apparel – etsy.com/shop/lizajanehandmade

Sweet potatoes are filled with antioxidants, anti-inflammatory nutrients, and blood sugar–regulating nutrients. These tasty, healthy fries should be added to everyone's diet.

BAKED SWEET POTATO FRIES

Serves 4

1 teaspoon salt
½ teaspoon pepper
1 teaspoon garlic powder
1 teaspoon onion powder
½ teaspoon paprika
1 teaspoon parsley
5 sweet potatoes, peeled and sliced into ¼-inch-long slices
olive oil for tossing

Preheat oven to 450 degrees F.

Combine salt, pepper, garlic powder, onion powder, paprika, and parsley and set seasoning aside.

Line a sheet tray with parchment. In a large bowl toss sweet potatoes with just enough oil to coat. Sprinkle with seasoning. Spread sweet potatoes in single layer on prepared baking sheet, being sure not to overcrowd.

Bake until sweet potatoes are tender and golden brown, turning occasionally, about 20 minutes. Serve hot.

"It is never too late to be who you might have been."
– ATTRIBUTED TO GEORGE ELIOT

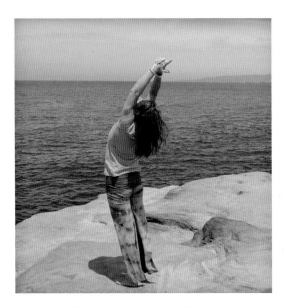

Outfit by Soul Flower – soul-flower.com
Bracelets by IndoLove – etsy.com/shop/IndoLove

UPWARD SALUTE

Begin in Mountain Pose (page 17) with your hands down at your sides. Inhale and sweep arms out and upward toward the ceiling. Press palms together firmly. Extend elbows and reach upward.

If you wish to add a gentle back bend, clasp your fingers, leaving your thumb and pointer finger straight. Gently tip head back and gaze at the sky. Lift rib cage away from your pelvis, opening up the belly.

Lengthen tail bone downward. Keep legs active, tailbone tucked, and core engaged. Keep adequate space between shoulders and ears. Hold for a few breaths.

Skip the chips and go for some spicy poppers. You can eat the whole bowl without any guilt!

CAULIFLOWER POPPERS

Serves 4

1½ teaspoons smoked paprika
½ teaspoon chili powder
½ teaspoon mesquite seasoning
1 teaspoon salt
½ teaspoon pepper
1 large head of cauliflower, cleaned and cut into pieces
2 tablespoons olive oil

Preheat oven to 425 degrees F. Line a baking sheet with aluminum foil or parchment paper.

In a small bowl mix the paprika, chili powder, mesquite seasoning, salt, and pepper together.

In another large bowl toss the cauliflower with the olive oil so that each piece is covered. Sprinkle the spices over the cauliflower pieces and toss to make sure each piece is coated with the spice mixture.

Place the cauliflower on the baking sheet and bake for 30 to 45 minutes or until golden brown. Turn every 15 minutes to ensure even browning.

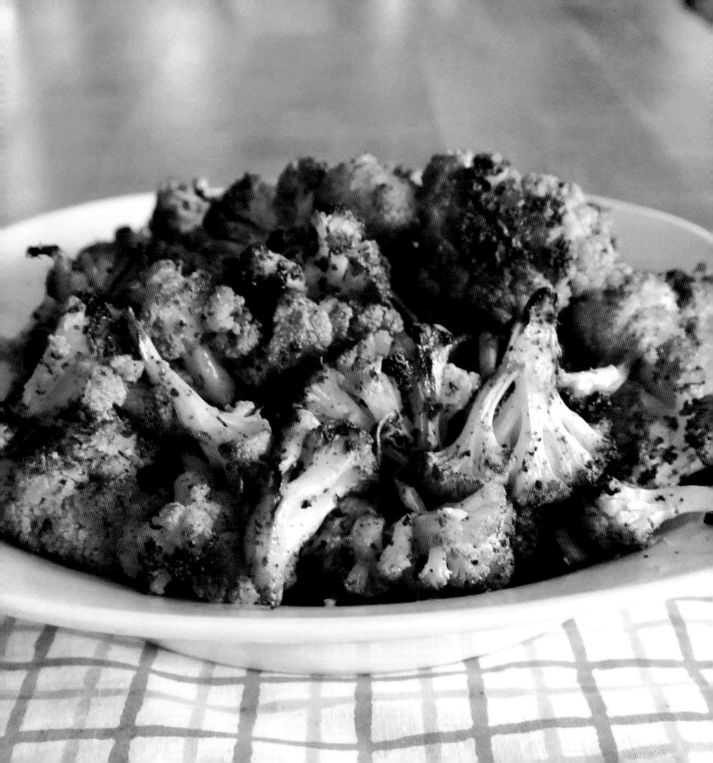

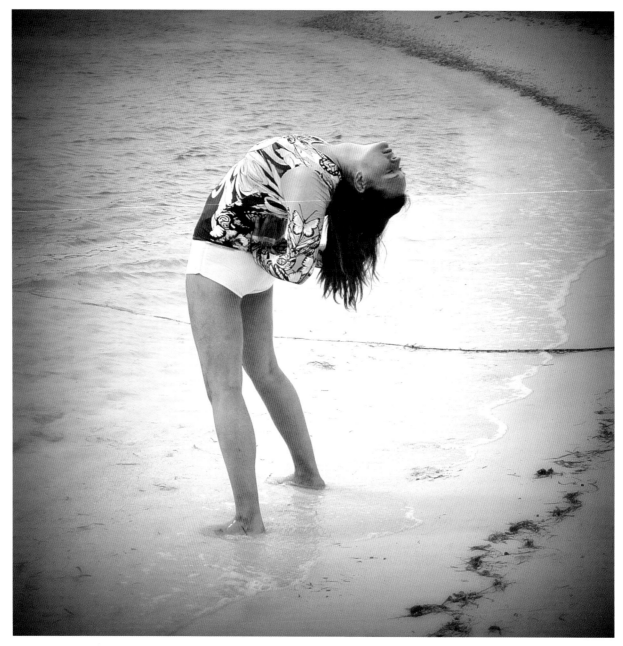

Top by YMX by Yellowman ymxbyyellowman.com
Shorts by Dragonfly dragonfly-yogawear.com

STANDING BACK BEND

From Mountain Pose (page 17), place the palms on the low back/sacrum with the fingers pointed down. Press into the feet, pull up the kneecaps, and squeeze the thighs and buttocks.

Press the hips forward and begin to arch the torso backwards. Keep the head looking forward, or if it feels safe let it drop all the way back. Use the arms to support your weight and keep the legs and buttocks engaged and strong.

"Let him who would move the world first move himself."
– ATTRIBUTED TO SOCRATES

Cauliflower helps me stick to my diet. Being oh-so-low in calories, only 27 calories for one cup of cauliflower, it is my go-to food. While everyone else munches on their potato chips, devour these healthy ones. Now my disclaimer is that they won't be as crunchy as potato chips unless you fry them. I don't fry them. I bake them until the outsides are crispy and the inside is a little chewy.

CAULIFLOWER RANCH CHIPS

Serves 4

1 cup grated Parmesan cheese
1 cup grated raw cauliflower
½ teaspoon parsley
½ teaspoon basil
½ teaspoon dill
½ teaspoon chives
½ teaspoon garlic powder
½ teaspoon onion powder
½ teaspoon pepper

Preheat oven to 450 degrees F. Add all ingredients to a bowl and stir.

Line a baking sheet or stone with parchment paper. Place about 1 tablespoon of mixture on prepared baking sheets, about 1 inch apart.

Bake at 450 degrees for 5–7 minutes. Remove and turn cauliflower chips over. Bake for another 5–7 minutes.

FORWARD FOLD

Begin in Mountain Pose (page 17) with your hands on your hips. Exhale as you bend forward at the hips, lengthening the front of your torso.

Bend your elbows and hold on to each elbow with the opposite hand. Let the crown of your head hang down. Press your heels into the floor as you lift your sit bones toward the ceiling. Turn the tops of your thighs slightly inward. Do not lock your knees.

If you can keep the front of your torso long and your knees straight, place your palms or fingertips on the floor beside your feet. Bring your fingertips in line with your toes and press your palms on the mat. Those with more flexibility can place their palms on the backs of their ankles or calves.

Engage your front thigh muscles and draw them up toward the ceiling. The more you engage your quadriceps, the more your rear thigh muscles will release.

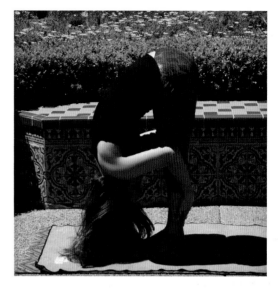

Outfit by Me and Harpua – etsy.com/shop/MeAndHarpua
Yoga Towel by EveryDay Yoga – etsy.com/shop/EverydayYoga

"Life is a great big canvas, and you should throw all the paint you can on it."
– DANNY KAYE

Adding almond meal to the coating adds protein and a crispy coating that we all crave.

CAULIFLOWER TOTS

Serves 4

2 eggs
⅓ cup rice flour
½ teaspoon garlic powder
½ teaspoon salt
¼ teaspoon pepper
½ cup crushed tortilla chips
½ cup ground almonds
1 head of raw cauliflower, grated
grapeseed oil or any high-temperature oil

Heat up a small skillet with oil, enough to cover a tot, over medium heat until it reaches 350 degrees F. Mix together eggs, rice flour, garlic powder, salt, and pepper until well-blended. In another bowl, add your crushed tortilla chips and ground almonds.

Blend well.

Create tater tot shapes with your hands by rolling the cauliflower dough into a ball, or if you have a 1-inch ring mold you can shape them that way, and then roll around each tot into the bread crumbs to completely coat.

Gently place the tots in batches (mine took 6 tots per batch) into the skillet with hot oil, and cook for about 3 minutes until lightly browned. Drain on a paper towel–lined plate. Serve warm with your favorite dipping sauce.

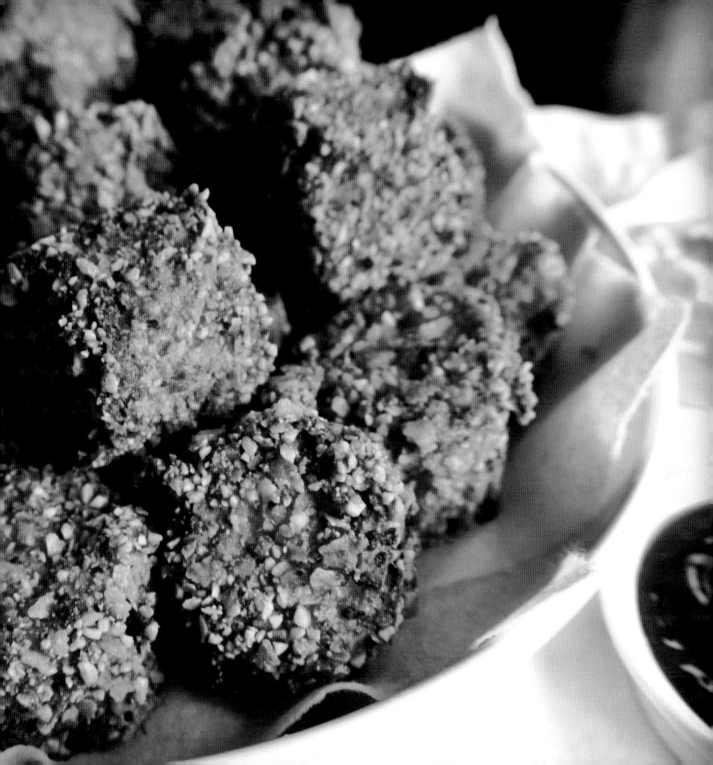

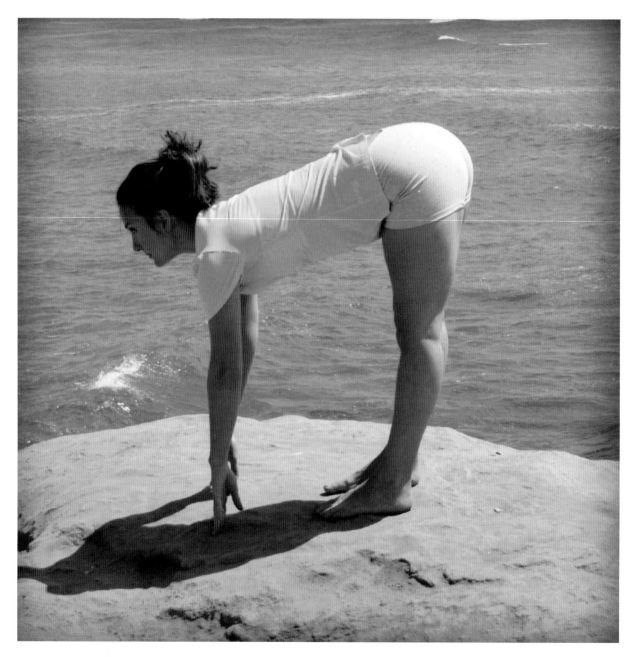

Outfit by Green Apple Activewear – greenappleactive.com

"Life is not measured by the number of breaths we take, but by the moments that
take our breath away."
– VICKI CORONA

HALFWAY LIFT

Face forward and bend to press your palms or fingertips into the floor in front of your feet. With an inhale, straighten your elbows and arch your torso away from your thighs, finding as much length between your pubic bone and navel as possible.

With your palms or fingertips, push down and back against the floor, and lift the top of your sternum up and forward. Look forward, but be careful not to compress the back of your neck.

With over 500,000 repins on Pinterest, this is by far my most popular healthy recipe to date. It is only fitting to include it in this book. It will knock your socks off!

GLUTEN-FREE, GRAIN-FREE CHEESY GARLIC CAULIFLOWER BREADSTICKS

Makes 12 sticks

small amount of olive oil
1 cup cooked cauliflower
1 egg, beaten
½ cup Parmesan cheese
½ cup shredded mozzarella cheese
1 teaspoon dried oregano
½ teaspoon crushed garlic
¼ teaspoon garlic salt

TOPPING:
2 tablespoons softened salted butter
2 cloves garlic, finely minced
¼ cup grated Parmesan cheese
¼ cup grated mozzarella cheese
optional marinara sauce for dipping

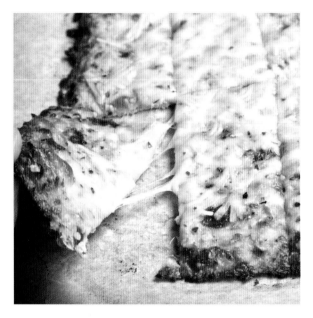

Preheat oven to 450 degrees F. Prepare your baking stone or sheet by spreading a small amount of olive oil on it and top with parchment paper. Rice the cooked cauliflower. You can do this in a ricer, or grate it, or process until fine in a food processor or blender. One large head should produce approximately 3 cups of riced cauliflower. The remainder can be used to make additional breadsticks immediately, or can be stored in the refrigerator for up to one week.

In a medium bowl, stir together cauliflower, egg, Parmesan cheese, and mozzarella cheese. Add oregano, crushed garlic, and garlic salt; stir. Transfer to the baking stone or sheet and, using your hands, pat out into a large rectangle.

Bake at 450 degrees for 15 minutes. Remove from oven. Mix 2 tablespoons butter and garlic in a small bowl and spread the butter and garlic mixture over baked cauliflower bread. Top with Parmesan and mozzarella cheeses. Place back in the 450-degree oven until all cheese is melted. Slice and serve!

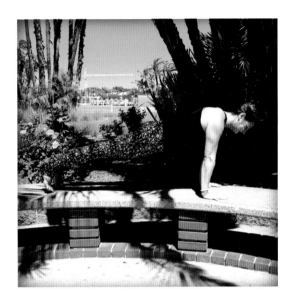

Top by Kira Grace – kiragrace.com
Leggings by Fractal9 – etsy.com/shop/Fractal9

"Smile, breathe, and go slowly."
– THICH NHAT HANH

PLANK POSE

Begin in Downward-Facing Dog Pose (page 43): arms straight, hands stable, fingers wide.

On the exhale, bring your body forward, lowering the hips and tailbone, making the back straight. Arms should be straight and the head and neck in line.

Push firmly away from the mat, not allowing shoulders, chest, or abdomen to sink; keep them firm and in line.

I like to add this to a bunch of super seeds to make a fabulous granola. With cocoa being a super food itself, you are simply making your granola extra super!

CHOCOLATE PROTEIN GRANOLA

Serves 6

2 cups rolled oats
½ cup dark chocolate chips
½ teaspoon cinnamon
½ cup raw mountain honey
1 tablespoon maple syrup
½ teaspoon vanilla extract
¼ cup melted coconut oil + extra for baking
¼ cup unsalted pumpkin seeds
¼ cup sunflower seeds
¼ cup sliced or whole almonds

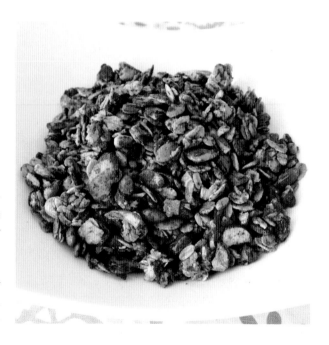

Preheat oven to 275 degrees F. Mix all dry ingredients in a bowl. Mix all liquid ingredients in a separate bowl. Combine all liquid and dry ingredients together in a large bowl, stirring evenly.

Place more coconut oil on a deep baking sheet. Slowly add the granola to the baking sheet and place in oven. Stir the granola every 15–20 minutes for even heat distribution for about 1 hour.

Remove from oven and let the melted chocolate settle in the granola and cool for 30 minutes.

You can munch on this plain for a snack, or eat it with almond milk for a meal. Store in an airtight container.

CHATARUNGA

Begin in Plank Pose (page 33). Keeping your elbows directly over your wrists, slowly lower your body to hover a few inches above the floor. Keep your back flat.

Lift through your chest, keeping your shoulders in line with your elbows. Do not let your chest drop or sag toward the floor.

Fully engage your abdominal and leg muscles. If the full pose is too challenging right now, come to your knees first. Then, lower your torso to hover an inch above the floor. Do not let your elbows splay to the sides. Keep them hugged along your rib cage, pointed toward your heels.

Press the base of your knuckles into the floor. Your upper and lower arms should be perpendicular, bent 90 degrees at the elbows. Do not let your shoulders drop lower than the height of your elbows.

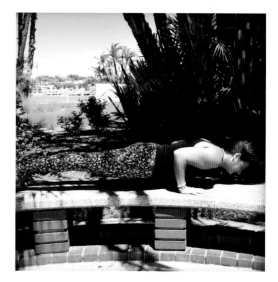

Top by Kira Grace – kiragrace.com
Leggings by Fractal9 – etsy.com/shop/fractal9

If veggies are an afterthought for you, try this simple crock-pot method. Then they are ready for you when you are hungry.

WHOLE ROASTED CAULIFLOWER

Serves 4

1 head of cauliflower
3 cloves garlic, crushed
2 tablespoons olive oil
1 tablespoon Italian seasoning or fresh herbs of your choice
1 cup chicken broth
salt and pepper to taste

Place all ingredients in the slow cooker and cook on low for 3–4 hours, until the cauliflower is tender. Salt and pepper to taste and serve.

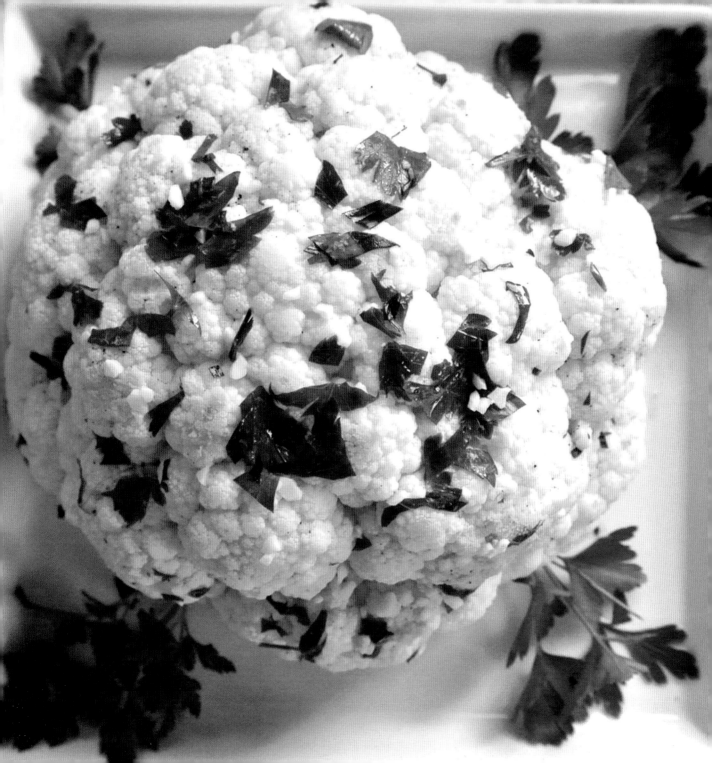

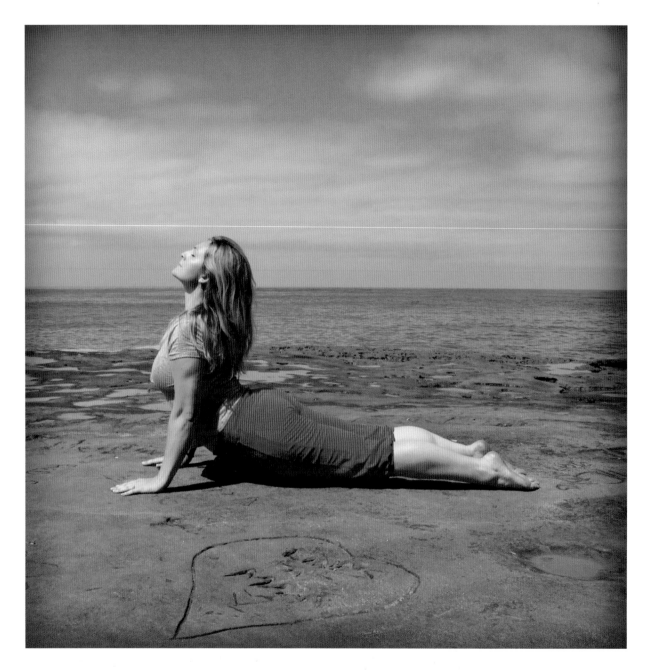

Outfit by Green Apple Activewear – greenappleactive.com

UPWARD-FACING DOG

Begin by lying face-down on the floor with your legs extended behind you, spread a few inches apart. The tops of your feet should rest on the mat.

Place your hands on the floor alongside your body, next to your lower ribs. Point your fingers to the top of the mat and hug your elbows in close to your ribs.

Inhale as you press through your hands firmly into the floor. Straighten your arms, lifting your torso and your legs a few inches off the floor.

Press down firmly through the tops of your feet. Strongly engage your leg muscles to keep your thighs lifted off the floor.

Keep your elbows pressed alongside your body. Drop your shoulders away from your ears and lift your chest toward the ceiling, drawing your shoulders back and your heart forward.

"Twenty years from now you will be more disappointed by the things you didn't do than by the ones you did do."
– H. JACKSON BROWN, JR.

I used to be sad watching others fill their faces with chips and salsa, until I realized I just needed to replace the crunch and I could enjoy it too. Eat the whole bowl without the guilt!

CUCUMBER CHIPS AND SALSA

Serves 4

½ sweet onion, diced
3 ripe tomatoes, diced
¼ cup chopped cilantro
2 garlic cloves, minced
1 jalapeño, diced (can add or reduce according to your heat preference)
salt and pepper to taste
2 cucumbers, peeled and sliced diagonally

In a small bowl, mix together the onion, tomatoes, cilantro, minced garlic, and jalapeño. Stir and add salt and pepper to taste.

Place your sliced cucumbers on a plate and top with salsa and serve. I garnish my plate with cilantro, but it is not necessary.

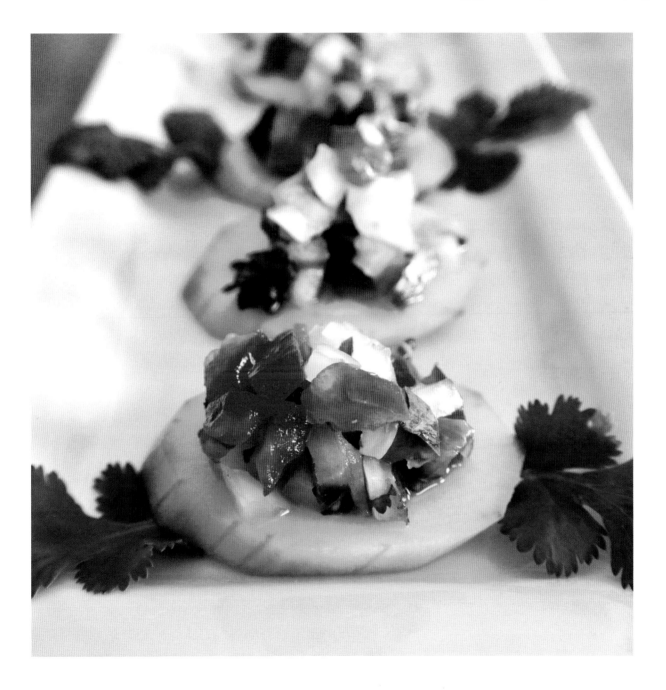

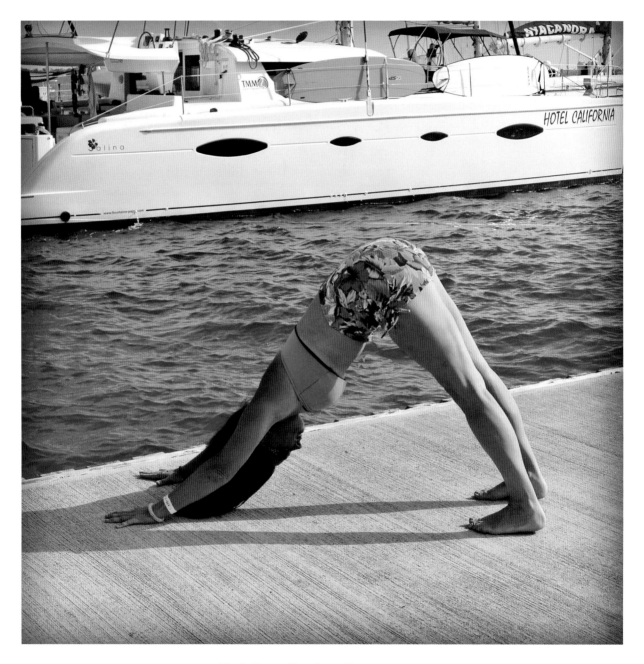

Top by Dragonfly – dragonfly-yogawear.com
Shorts by Fractal9 – etsy.com/shop/Fractal9

"What lies behind us and what lies before us are tiny matters compared to what lies within us."
– RALPH WALDO EMERSON

DOWNWARD-FACING DOG

Begin on your hands and knees in a tabletop position. Align your wrists directly under your shoulders and your knees directly under your hips. The fold of your wrists should be parallel with the top edge of your mat.

Spread your fingers out wide and press firmly through your palms and fingers, distributing your weight evenly across your hands.

Tuck your toes, exhale, and lift your knees off the floor. Reach your pelvis up toward the ceiling, then draw your sit bones back behind you. Gently begin to straighten your legs.

Press the floor away from you as you lift through your pelvis, being sure not to lock your knees. As you lengthen your spine, lift your sit bones up toward the sky. Now press down equally through your heels and the palms of your hands.

Firm the outer muscles of your arms and press your index fingers into the floor. Lift from the inner muscles of your arms to the top of both shoulders. Draw your shoulder blades into your upper back ribs and toward your tailbone.

Rotate your arms externally so your elbow creases face your thumbs.

Draw your chest toward your thighs as you continue to press the mat away from you, lengthening and decompressing your spine.

Engage your quadriceps. Rotate your thighs inward as you continue to lift your sit bones high. Sink your heels toward the floor.

Align your ears with your upper arms. Relax your head, but do not let it dangle. Gaze between your legs or toward your navel.

Eliminating mayonnaise makes these scrumptious deviled eggs guilt-free; two eggs are only 83 calories. That makes them a great healthy snack or appetizer.

HEALTHIER DEVILED EGGS

Serves 4

8 large eggs, hard-boiled and peeled
¼ cup plain Greek yogurt
1 tablespoon vinegar
1 tablespoon mustard
¼ teaspoon sea salt
⅛ teaspoon pepper
paprika for garnishing

Halve hard-boiled eggs lengthwise. Remove yolks and place in a small bowl.

Whisk together yolks, Greek yogurt, vinegar, mustard, salt, and pepper. Fill egg whites evenly with yolk mixture. Sprinkle with paprika and serve.

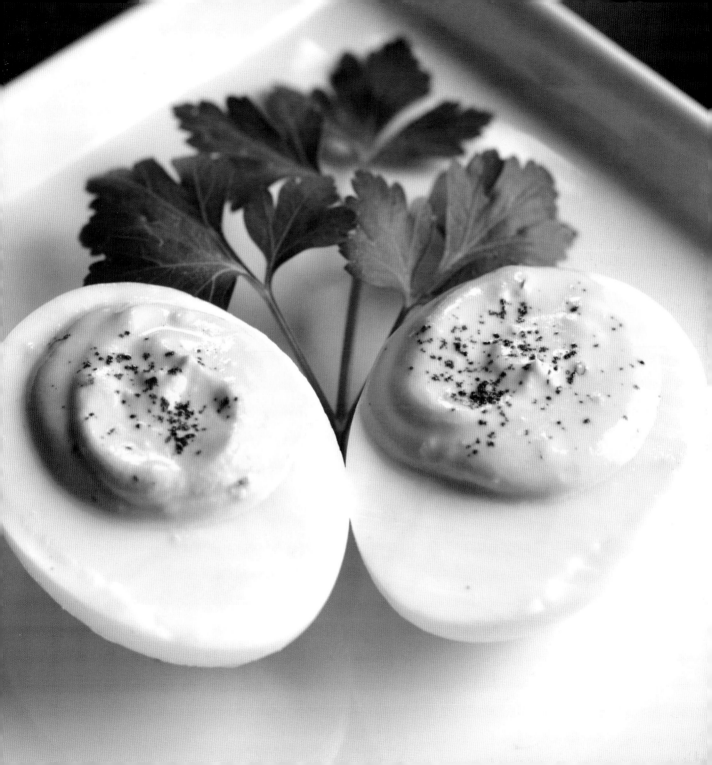

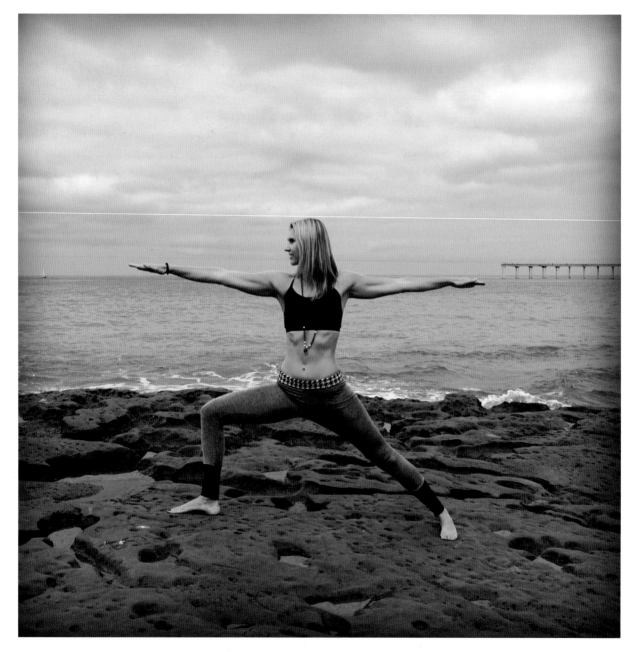

Outfit by Proper Fit – etsy.com/shop/ProperFit
Necklace by Indo Love Jewelry – etsy.com/shop/IndoLove

WARRIOR 2

Begin in a lunge with your right foot forward, toes pointed forward, and left foot back with toes turned slightly out (at a 45-degree angle). Align your front heel with the arch of your back foot.

Deepen the lunge, keeping your front knee stacked over your front ankle. Straighten your back leg. The back edge of your back foot is your anchor for this pose; firmly press down for more stability.

Extend your arms, pushing your energy out of your fingertips as you gaze towards your front fingers.

"Whatever you do, you should do it with feeling."
– YOGI BERRA

This is my all-time go-to summer drink. I keep frozen organic fruit in my freezer year-round for a quick meal replacement solution.

GREEN PIÑA COLADA

Serves 1

¾ cup fresh orange juice
1 cup frozen pineapple
1 avocado, peeled, pit removed, and sliced
1 frozen banana
½ cup coconut milk

Place all ingredients in your blender and blend until smooth. Serve immediately.

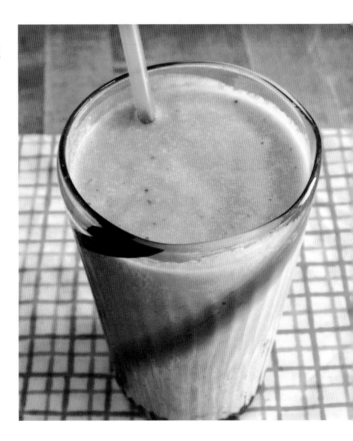

EXTENDED SIDE ANGLE

Begin in Mountain Pose (page 17). Turn to the left and extend your arms sideways to shoulder-height, palms facing down. Step your feet as wide apart as your wrists.

Turn your right leg and foot outward 90 degrees so your toes point to the top of your mat. Bend your right knee until your right thigh is as parallel as you can get it to the floor. Keep your right knee directly over your heel. Turn in your left toes slightly. Align the heel of your right foot with the arch of your left foot. Keep your back leg straight. Inhale and draw your left hip slightly forward.

Exhaling, lower your right arm reaching for the ground next to your front foot.

Reach your left arm up towards the ceiling, and then extend your arm over the top of your head. Your left biceps should be over your left ear, and your fingertips should be reaching in the same direction your front toes are pointing. Keep your chest, hips, and legs in one straight line, extended over your front leg.

Turn your head to look up at the ceiling. Keep your throat soft and your breathing smooth. Relax your face.

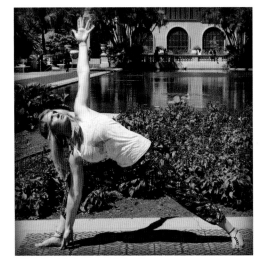

Top By Think Positive Apparel – thinkpositiveapparel.com
Pants by Mogul Interior – mogulinterior.com
Barefoot Sandals by Anchro – etsy.com/shop/Anchro

"Success each day should be judged by the seeds sown, not the harvest reaped."
– JOHN C. MAXWELL

Ranch does not have to be bad for you. Using Greek yogurt, you can have all the taste without any of the guilt.

GREEK RANCH DIP

Serves 4

1 cup plain Greek yogurt
2 tablespoons white vinegar
2 large garlic cloves, smashed and finely minced (about 2 heaping teaspoons)
2 tablespoons finely chopped green onions
2 tablespoons chopped chives
¼ cup minced Italian parsley
½ teaspoon chopped fresh thyme leaves
coarse salt and freshly ground black pepper to taste

Mix together. Chill until you serve.

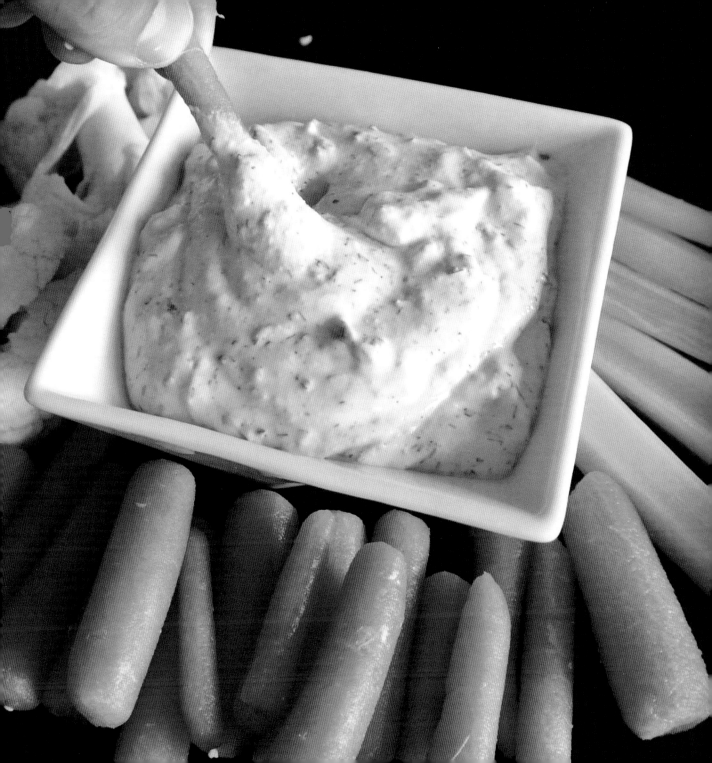

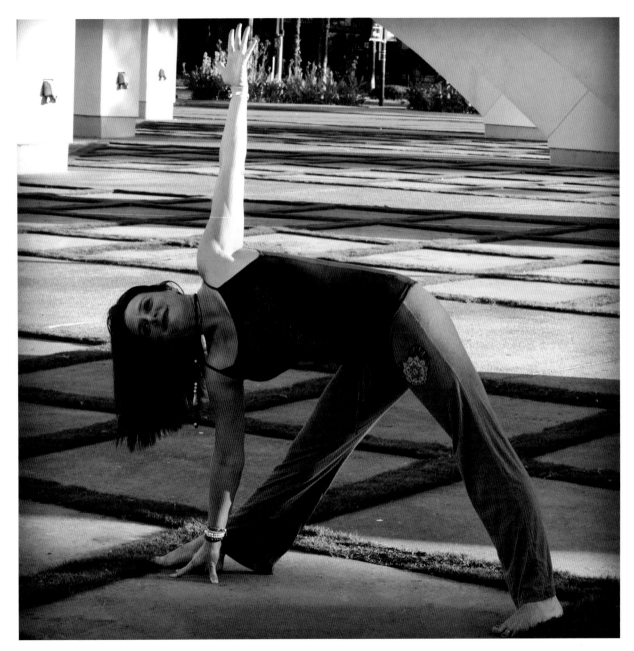

Outfit by Soul Flower – soul-flower.com
Necklace by True Nature Jewelry – etsy.com/shop/TrueNatureJewelry
Bracelets by Indo Love Jewelry – etsy.com/shop/IndoLove

TRIANGLE POSE

Begin standing. Keep your feet wide apart (4 to 5 feet).

Turn your right foot out 90 degrees so your toes are pointing to the top of the mat. The center of your right kneecap should be aligned with the center of your right ankle.

Pivot your left foot slightly inwards. Your back toes should be at a 45-degree angle. Your right heel should align with the arch of your left foot. Lift through the arches of your feet while rooting down through your ankles.

Raise your arms at your sides to shoulder-height, so they're parallel to the floor. Your arms should be aligned directly over your legs. With your palms facing down, reach actively from fingertip to fingertip.

On an exhalation, reach through your right hand in the same direction as your right foot is pointed. Shift your left hip back so your tailbone and pelvis tilt toward the wall or space behind your left foot. Fold at your right hip. Keep your right ear, shoulder, and knee on the same plane. Turn your left palm forward, with your fingertips reaching toward the sky.

Rest your right hand on your outer shin, ankle, or the ground, but maintain muscular energy in both arms.

"The results you achieve will be in direct proportion to the effort you apply."
– DENIS WAITLEY

Avocados contain healthy fat your body needs to function. This is a fabulous healthy snack or appetizer full of nutrients.

GUACAMOLE

Serves 4

1 cup diced sweet onion
4 garlic cloves, minced
4 serrano chiles, minced
juice of 2 limes
6 ripe avocados
sea salt to taste

Put the onion, garlic, chiles, lime juice, and avocados in a bowl.

Use a large serving fork and mix up the ingredients. Then, press the fork around the sides of the bowl to mas the avocados. This will make a chunky guacamole.

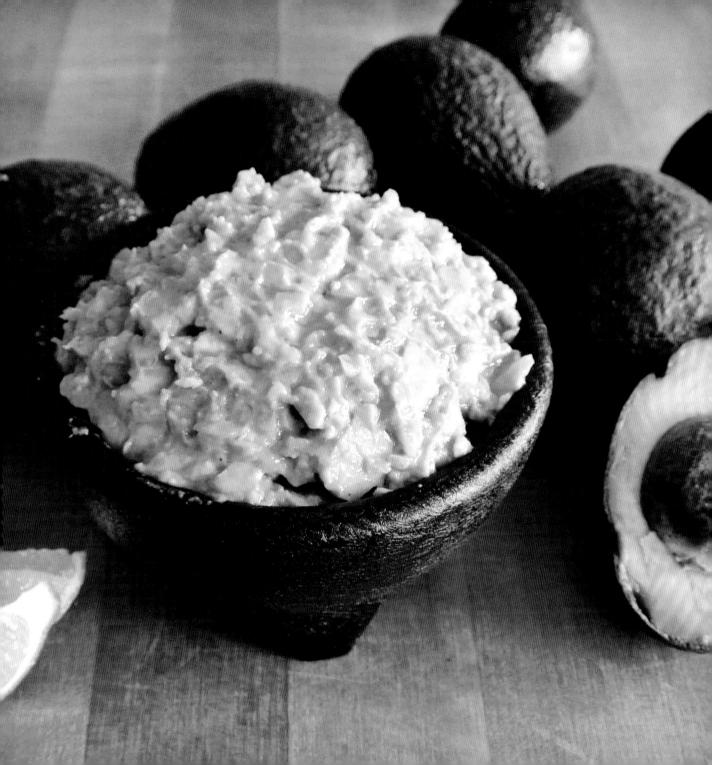

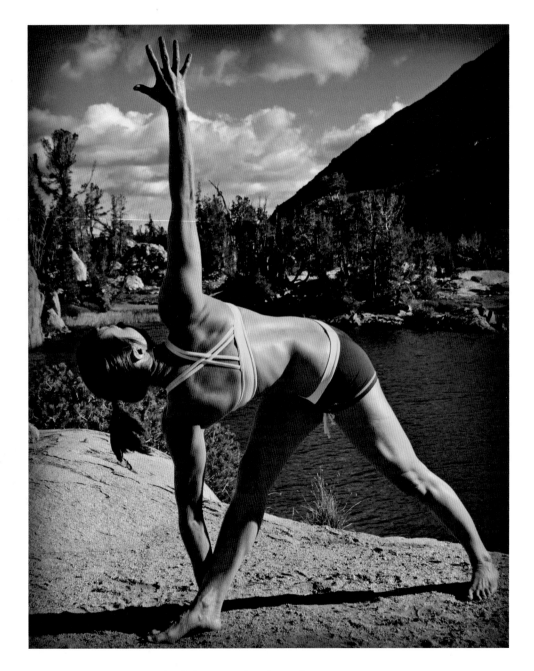

Outfit by Dragonfly – dragonfly-yogawear.com

REVOLVED TRIANGLE POSE

Begin in Mountain Pose (page 17). Turn your right foot out 90 degrees so your toes are pointing to the top of the mat. The center of your right kneecap should be aligned with the center of your right ankle. Pivot your left foot inward to a 45-degree angle.

Bring your hands to your hips and square your hips forward.

Raise your left arm toward the ceiling, with your biceps next to your left ear. Reach up strongly through your left hand.

On an exhalation, hinge forward from your hips, keeping your spine long. Place your left hand to the outside of your right foot as you open your torso to the right.

Use your right hand to draw your right hip back so it stays in line with your left hip.

Inhale and lengthen your spine again. Then, exhale as you roll your right shoulder back and extend your right arm straight up toward the ceiling.

Reach strongly through your right fingertips. Turn your head to gaze at your right thumb.

"Winners compare their achievements with their goals, while losers compare their achievements with those of other people."
– NIDO QUBEIN

Parsnips are a great healthy alternative to potatoes, and when cooked like this, they taste just like potatoes au gratin, but are much healthier.

PARSNIP GRATIN

Serves 4

olive oil
2 cups plain Greek yogurt
½ cup whole milk
1¼ teaspoons kosher salt
¼ teaspoon fresh ground nutmeg
¼ teaspoon pepper
1 tablespoon fresh minced thyme
3 large minced cloves of garlic
2¼ pounds parsnips, peeled and sliced into ⅛-inch-thick slices
1 medium onion, diced
6 ounces grated sharp cheddar cheese

Preheat oven to 400 degrees F. Generously grease a 6 × 9–inch baking dish with olive oil. In a bowl, add Greek yogurt, milk, salt, nutmeg, pepper, thyme, and garlic. Stir. This is your cream mixture.

Put a solid layer of the parsnips in the bottom of the prepared pan.

Top parsnip layer with onion and a layer of the cream mixture, and a layer of the grated cheese. Keep repeating these two steps until all the ingredients are used up.

Cover securely with a lid or foil and bake for 50 minutes on the middle rack. Serve.

WIDE-LEGGED FORWARD FOLD

Begin in Mountain Pose (page 17). Turn to the left and extend your arms sideways to shoulder-height, palms facing down. Step your feet as wide apart as your wrists.

Turn your right leg and foot outward 90 degrees so your toes point to the top of your mat. Bend your right knee until your right thigh is as parallel as you can get it to the floor. Keep your right knee directly over your heel. Turn in your left toes slightly. Align the heel of your right foot with the arch of your left foot. Keep your back leg straight. Inhale and draw your left hip slightly forward.

Exhaling, lower your right arm, reaching for the ground next to your front foot.

Reach your left arm up towards the ceiling, and then extend your arm over the top of your head. Your left biceps should be over your left ear, and your fingertips should be reaching in the same direction your front toes are pointing. Keep your chest, hips, and legs in one straight line, extended over your front leg.

Turn your head to look up at the ceiling. Keep your throat soft and your breathing smooth. Relax your face.

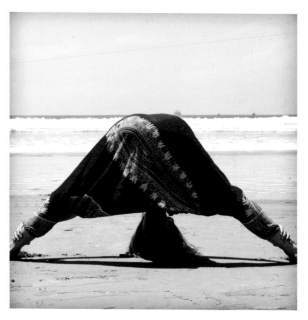

Pants by Mogul Interior – mogulinterior.com

A big step in eating healthy is learning to substitute quinoa for rice and potatoes as much as possible. Here is a fast recipe for perfect quinoa every time.

PERFECTLY COOKED QUINOA

Makes 2 cups cooked quinoa

1 cup quinoa
2 cups filtered water

Bring water to a boil. Add quinoa, cover, and put heat on low for 20 minutes. Don't open the lid. It will be perfect in 20 minutes. You can add salt if you wish, but I use quinoa for both sweet and savory dishes, so I just season mine later according to the recipe I am using.

Quinoa keeps nicely in the fridge in an airtight container for 5 days.

REVERSE WARRIOR

Begin in a lunge with your right foot forward, toes pointed forward, and left foot back, toes turned slightly out at a 45-degree angle. Align your front heel with the arch of your back foot.

Deepen the lunge, keeping your front knee stacked over your front ankle. Straighten your back leg. The back edge of your back foot is your anchor for this pose; firmly press down for more stability.

On your exhalation, place your back hand on the back of your left thigh. On an inhalation, lift your right arm straight up, and then reach your fingertips towards the wall behind you. Your right biceps should be next to your right ear.

Keep your front knee bent and your hips sinking low as you lengthen through the sides of your waist. Slide your back hand further down your leg and come into a graceful side bend. Gaze at your fingertips in the sky.

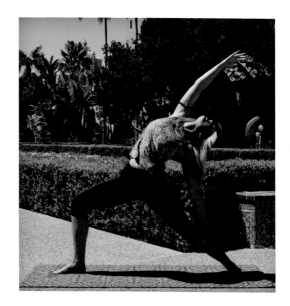

Outfit by Onzie – onzie.com

"Don't think, just do."
– ATTRIBUTED TO HORACE

I have found the solution to snacking is having foods on hand that crunch. Get ready for a new addiction; these are so tasty!

PICKLED GREEN BEANS

Serves 4

1½ cup distilled white vinegar
¼ cup kosher salt
1½ cup hot water
2 heads fresh dill weed
4 garlic cloves
4 red Thai chile peppers (bird's eye chiles)
1¼ cup fresh green beans, washed and trimmed

Combine the water, salt, and vinegar in a large pot and bring to a boil. When it begins to boil, reduce heat to low and keep at a simmer. Meanwhile, pack the jars with dill weed, garlic cloves, Thai pepper and green beans into jars.

Pour the water/vinegar/salt mixture into the packed jars.

Close the airtight jar and store in the fridge. The beans will keep in the refrigerator for two months—if they don't get eaten first.

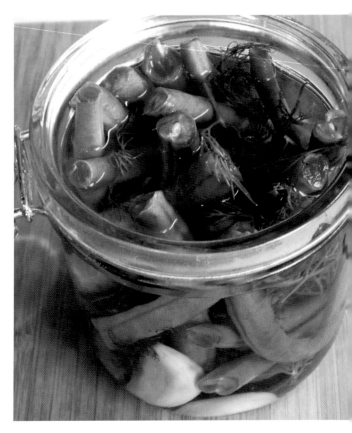

BACKBEND

Lay on the ground. Plant your feet firmly on the ground and bend your knees at a 90-degree angle. Put your palms by the sides of your head. Your fingers should be facing your feet. Point your elbows toward the ceiling.

When you're in position, gently push off the ground with your hands while keeping your hands and feet planted. Push off each hand at the same time and with the same force.

Keep pushing until your arms are straight and your legs are only a little bit bent. Your gaze should fall between your hands. You should be pushing with your finger pads and palms, taking the pressure off your wrists.

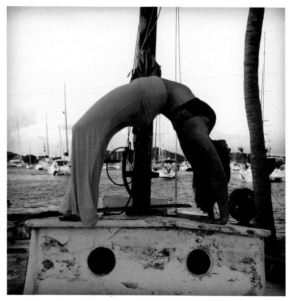

Top by Paramita Flow Designs – etsy.com/shop/paramitaflowdesigns
Pants by Liza and Jane Handmade – etsy.com/shop/lizajanehandmade

"If the world seems cold to you, kindle fires to warm it."
– LUCY LARCOM

Be careful buying packaged kale chips at the store. A lot of them are full of bad non-food ingredients and powders. These are simple to make at home and a great snack!

RANCH KALE CHIPS

Serves 4

1 head kale, washed and thoroughly dried
2 tablespoons olive oil
2 tablespoons parsley
2 teaspoons garlic powder
2 teaspoons onion powder
1½ teaspoons dill
1 teaspoon salt
½ teaspoon pepper

Preheat the oven to 275 degrees F. Remove the ribs from the kale and discard.

Cut kale leaves into bite size pieces. Toss kale with olive oil, parsley, garlic powder, onion powder, dill, salt, and pepper. I find it easiest to put in a large zip-lock bag and add the ingredients, then shake it.

Lay on a baking sheet and bake until crisp, about 20–25 minutes; turn leaves halfway through. Serve immediately or store in an airtight container.

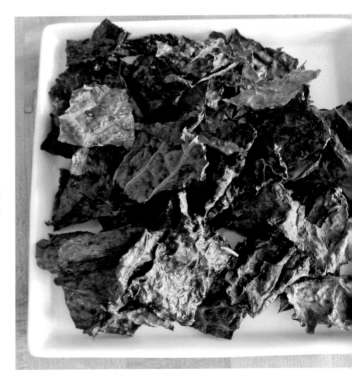

HALF MOON POSE

Begin in Revolved Triangle Pose (page 57) Bring your left hand to rest on your left hip. Turn your head to look at the floor. Then, bend your right knee and step your left foot 6–12 inches closer to your right foot. Place your right hand's fingertips on the floor in front of your right foot.

Press firmly into your right hand and foot. Straighten your right leg while simultaneously lifting your left leg. Work toward bringing your left leg parallel to the floor, or even higher than your hips.

Reach actively through your left heel. Do not lock your right knee. Keep your right toes and kneecap facing in the direction of your head.

Stack your top hip directly over your bottom hip, and open your torso to the left. Then, extend your left arm and point your fingertips directly toward the sky. If you can balance comfortably there, turn your head and gaze at your left thumb.

Draw your shoulder blades firmly into your back. Lengthen your tailbone toward your left heel.

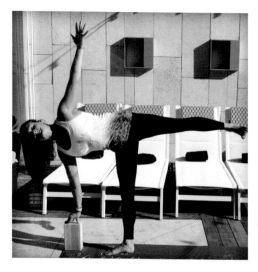

Top by My Positive Vibes – mypositivevibes.com
Leggings by DOV Clothing – dovclothing.com

"If your actions inspire others to dream more, learn more, do more, and become more, you are a leader."
– DOLLY PARTON

There is always time for vegetables. These come together in less than 10 minutes!

SAUTÉED VEGETABLES

Serves 4

3 tablespoons olive oil
1 large onion, thinly sliced in half-circles
2 cloves garlic, sliced
2 small zucchini, sliced
1 red pepper, sliced
1 yellow pepper, sliced
1 green pepper, sliced
½ teaspoon sea salt
⅛ teaspoon freshly ground black pepper
½ teaspoon dried oregano

Heat oil in a skillet set over medium heat. Add onion and garlic; sauté for about 3 minutes or until translucent.

Stir in zucchini, peppers, and spices. Cook, stirring occasionally, for 5–7 minutes or until tender-crisp.

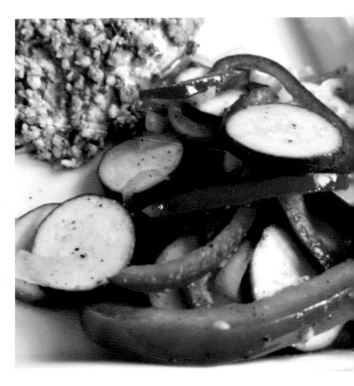

CHAIR POSE

Begin in Mountain Pose (page 17). Inhale and raise your arms above your head, perpendicular to the floor.

Exhale as you bend your knees, bringing your thighs as parallel to the floor as they can get without having your knees go past your toes.

Draw your shoulder blades into your upper back ribs as you reach your elbows back towards your ears. Draw your tailbone down to the floor, keeping your lower back long.

Shift your weight into your heels, enough that you could lift your toes if you want to.

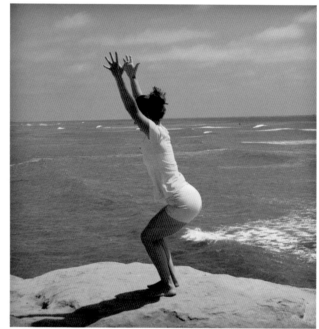

Outfit by Green Apple Activewear – greenappleactive.com

"Never leave that till tomorrow which you can do today."
– BENJAMIN FRANKLIN

Subbing parsnips for potatoes changes the nutrition value, not the taste or texture.

SHOESTRING GARLIC PARSNIP FRIES

Serves 4

2 large parsnips
1 teaspoon sea salt
½ teaspoon pepper
1 teaspoon garlic powder
½ teaspoon onion powder
1 teaspoon fresh, chopped parsley
2 tablespoons olive oil

Preheat the oven to 375 degrees F. Peel the parsnips as you would carrots. Slice into long strips (about ⅓-inch thick).

Mix all the salt and spices together. Toss with olive oil (about 1 tablespoon per 1 large parsnip) and sprinkle with the seasoning mixture.

Line a baking sheet, pan, or stone with parchment paper. Lay out your parsnips, being careful not to overlap them. If you overlap, they won't get crispy. Roast for 30 to 40 minutes, tossing in the middle, until you get browned edges.

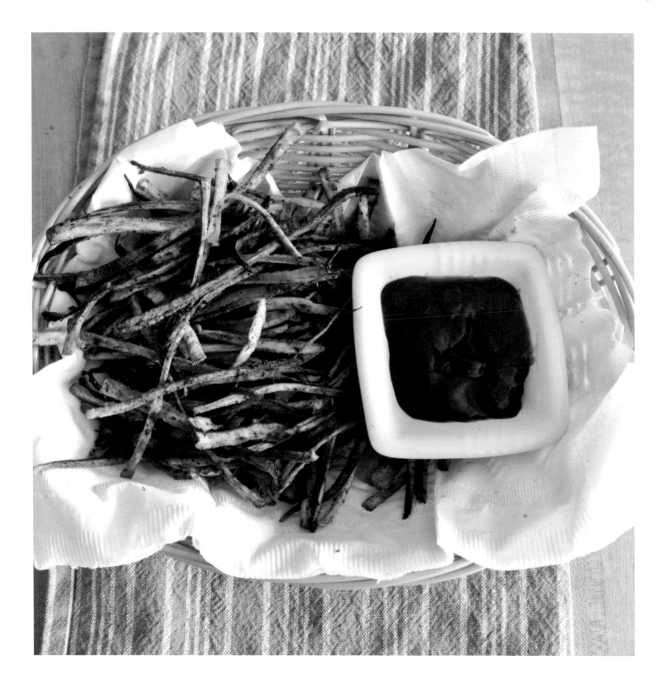

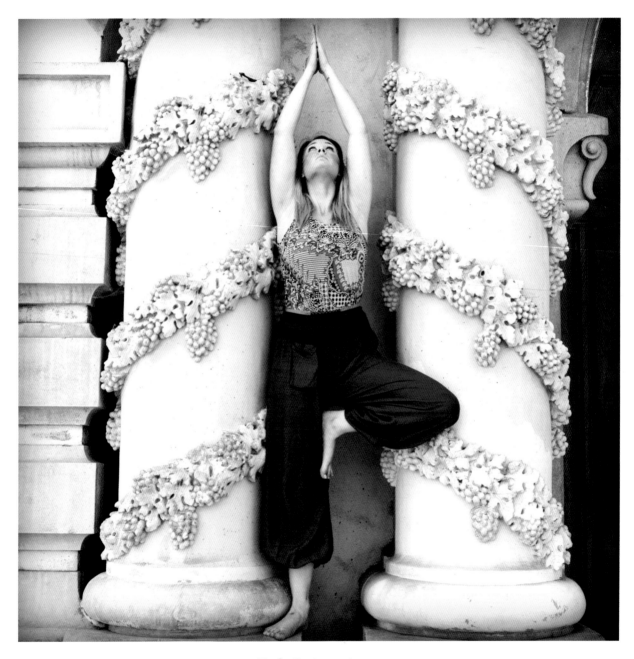

Top by Onzie – onzie.com
Pants by The High Thai – thehighthai.com

> "The price of discipline is always less than the pain of regret."
> **– NIDO QUBEIN**

TREE POSE

Begin by standing with your arms at your sides. Distribute your weight evenly across both feet, grounding down equally through your inner ankles, outer ankles, big toes, and baby toes.

Shift your weight to your left foot. Bend your right knee, then reach down and clasp your right inner ankle. Use your hand to draw your right foot alongside your inner left thigh. Do not rest your foot against your knee, only above or below it. Adjust your position so the center of your pelvis is directly over your left foot. Then, adjust your hips so your right hip and left hip are aligned.

Rest your hands on your hips and lengthen your tailbone toward the floor. Then, press your palms together in prayer position at your chest, with your thumbs resting on your sternum.

Draw down through your left foot. Press your right foot into your left thigh, while pressing your thigh equally against your foot.

Inhale as you extend your arms overhead, reaching your fingertips to the sky. Rotate your palms inward to face each other. If your shoulders are more flexible, you can press your palms together in prayer position, overhead. If steady, move your gaze slowly upward. Remember to repeat on the other leg.

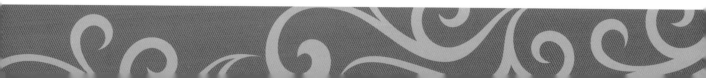

I like to put this slaw on sandwiches, wraps, and garden burgers. Or just eat a big bowl à la carte.

SPICY ASIAN SLAW

Serves 4

⅓ cup canola oil
⅓ cup fish sauce
¼ cup fresh lime juice
¼ cup rice vinegar
1 tablespoon sugar
1 tablespoon chopped garlic
1 chopped serrano pepper
2 tablespoons chopped fresh mint
1 head cabbage, cored and shredded
2 cups grated carrots

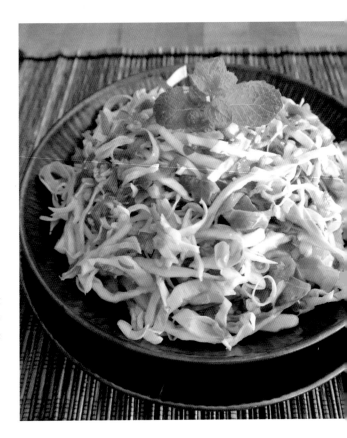

Mix first 7 ingredients together and whisk well.

Toss together mint, cabbage, and carrots. Pour wet ingredients over and toss. Refrigerate until ready to use. I stir mine every 30 minutes or so to make sure the flavors are well distributed. Strain prior to serving.

TWISTED CHAIR

Begin in Mountain Pose (page 17). On your inhale, come into Chair Pose (page 67). With big toes and inner thighs touching, bend at the knees, lower the hips and tailbone, eliminating the arching from the lower back, and shift the shins back to encourage the weight into the heels.

With hands together at the heart, twist to the right on the exhalation, hooking the left elbow to the outside of the right thigh, coming into side prayer twist or Twisted Chair.

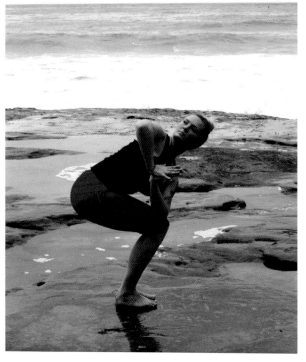

Outfit by Hotdrop – hotdrop.com

"The secret of getting ahead is getting started."
– ATTRIBUTED TO AGATHA CHRISTIE

I use these as a replacement for hash browns or potatoes. Potatoes make me sleepy, but quinoa gives me energy. Try this tasty replacement!

SPICY QUINOA CAKES

Makes 8 patties

2 cups cooked quinoa, at room temperature (leftover quinoa is perfect)
3 large eggs
½ teaspoon fine-grain sea salt
⅓ cup finely chopped fresh chives
1 small sweet onion, finely chopped
⅓ cup freshly grated pepper jack cheese
2 cloves garlic, finely chopped
½ teaspoon cayenne pepper
¼ cup crushed tortilla chips
1 tablespoon extra virgin olive oil

Combine the quinoa, eggs, and salt in a medium bowl and mix well. Stir in the chives, onion, cheese, garlic, and pepper. Add the tortilla chips, stir well, and then let the mixture rest for a few minutes.

Form the mixture into thick patties. Heat the oil in a large, heavy skillet over medium heat until simmering, swirling to thoroughly coat the bottom of the pan. Working in batches, gently place patties in the pan, leaving space between for easy flipping.

Cover and cook for 5 minutes, until the bottoms are browned. Carefully flip the patties with a spatula and cook the other sides for 4 minutes or until golden. Remove patties from the skillet and cool on a wire rack while you cook the remaining patties.

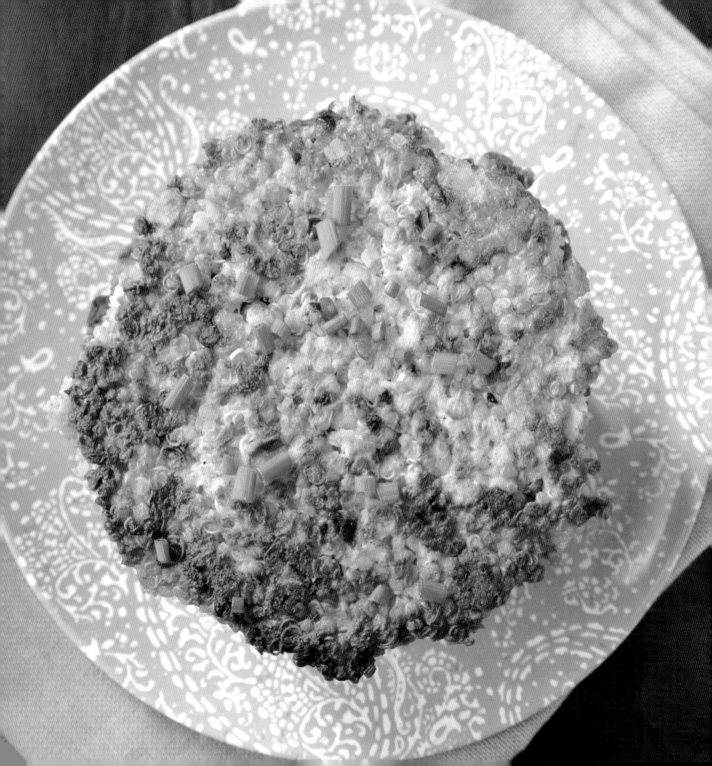

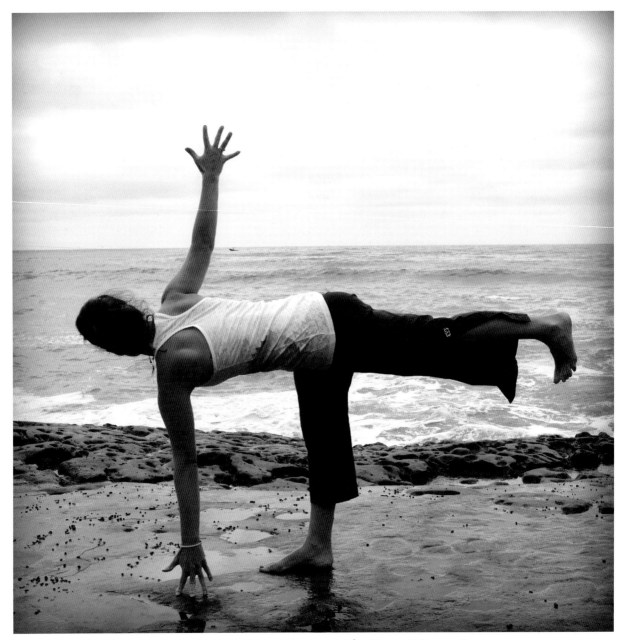

Top by Cocoon by Suzanne B – etsy.com/shop/CocoonBySuzanneB
Pants by Be Present – bepresent.com
Bracelet by IndoLove – etsy.com/shop/IndoLove

"To move the world we must first move ourselves."
– SOCRATES

REVOLVED HALF MOON

Begin in Revolved Triangle Pose (page 57). Lower your left hand and rest it on your left hip. Turn your head to look at the floor. Bend your right knee and step your left foot about 6–12 inches closer to your right foot. Place your right hand's fingertips on the floor in front of your right foot. Press firmly into your right hand and right foot.

Lift your left leg while simultaneously straightening your right leg. Bring your left leg parallel to the floor and reach actively through your left heel. Stack your top hip over your bottom hip and open your torso to the left. Extend your left arm and reach your fingertips to the sky. Gaze at your left thumb. You know this as Half Moon Pose (page 65).

Turn your gaze back to the floor. Lower your left hip so it's in line with your right hip. At the same time, bring your left hand to the floor in front of your right foot. Both front hips should now be facing the floor, and your lower back should be flat. Point your left foot's toes straight down toward the floor.

Bring your right hand to your right hip. Realign your hips so they are both parallel to the floor. You might need to draw your right hip slightly back.

Lift strongly through your left leg. Make sure your right foot's toes and right kneecap are pointing directly toward the top of your mat

Extend your spine from the tailbone through the crown of your head. Turn your upper torso to the right, twisting around your spine.

Reach your right arm up toward the ceiling. Turn your head and gaze up at your right thumb.

Mornings can be hard. Keeping organic frozen fruit in your freezer can lend to easy, quick, healthy smoothies that come together in under 5 minutes.

STRAWBERRY CITRUS SMOOTHIE

Serves 1

½ cup almond milk
½ cup plain Greek yogurt
½ cup fresh-squeezed orange juice
1 frozen banana
1 cup frozen strawberries
1 teaspoon chia seeds

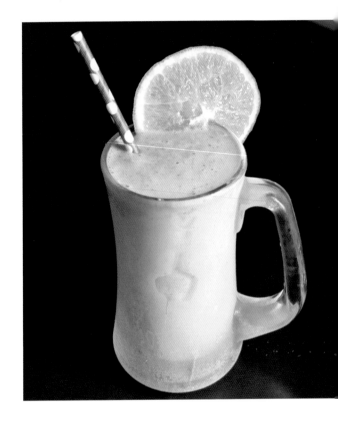

Add all ingredients to a blender and blend until it forms a milkshake consistency. Serve immediately.

EAGLE POSE

Stand in Mountain Pose (page 17). Bend your knees slightly, lift your left foot up, and, balancing on your right foot, cross your left thigh over the right. Point your left toes toward the floor, press the foot back, and then hook the top of the foot behind the lower right calf. Balance on the right foot.

Stretch your arms straight forward, parallel to the floor. Cross your arms in front of your torso so that the right arm is above the left, then bend your elbows. Snug the right elbow into the crook of the left, and raise the forearms perpendicular to the floor. The backs of your hands should be facing each other.

Press the right hand to the right and the left hand to the left, so that the palms are now facing each other. The thumb of the right hand should pass in front of the little finger of the left. Now press the palms together as much as is possible, lift your elbows up, and stretch the fingers toward the sky. Remember to repeat on the opposite side too.

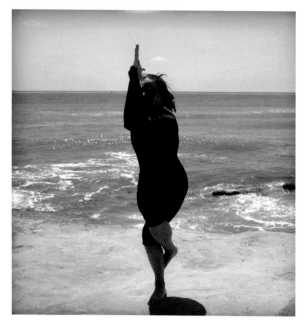

Top by YMX by Yellowman – ymxbyyellowman.com
Leggings by Green Apple Activewear – greenappleactive.com

"Well done is better than well said."
– BENJAMIN FRANKLIN

Here is a wholesome way to enjoy a wrap or sandwich. Every ingredient matters and is good for your body. Serve with everything you would serve with mayo. Veggie wraps are my favorite, but tuna salad is a close second.

VEGAN CASHEW MAYONNAISE

Makes 1 jar

1 cup cashews
2 tablespoon lemon juice
¼ cup vegetable broth
4 tablespoons water
salt to taste

Put one cup of raw cashews in a bowl and cover them with water. Let them sit for a minimum of 2 hours (up to overnight if you wish).

Drain and rinse the cashews, then pop them in your blender or food processor with 2 tablespoons of freshly squeezed lemon juice, ¼ cup of vegetable broth, and 4 tablespoons water.

Blend everything until it's completely smooth, scraping down the sides of the blender or food processor as needed. Salt to taste.

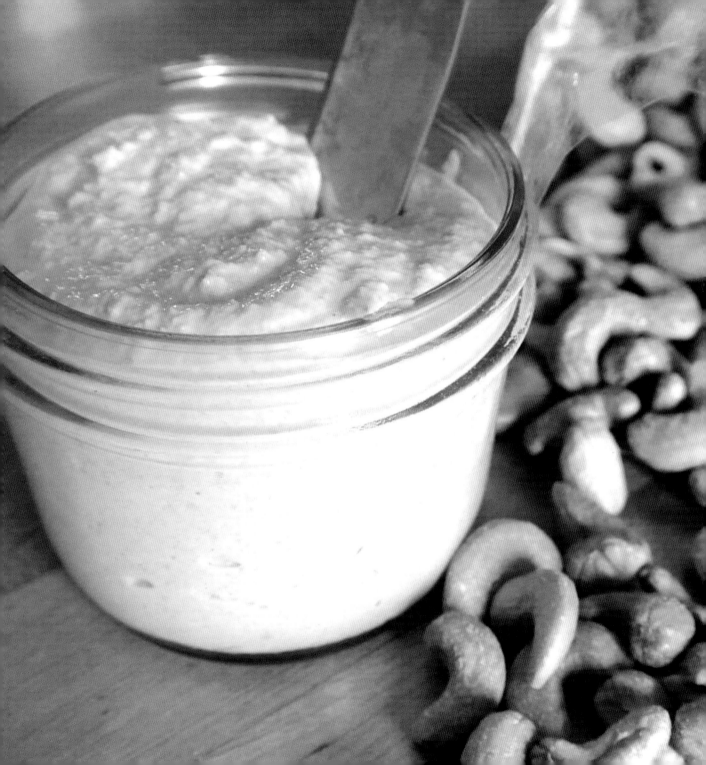

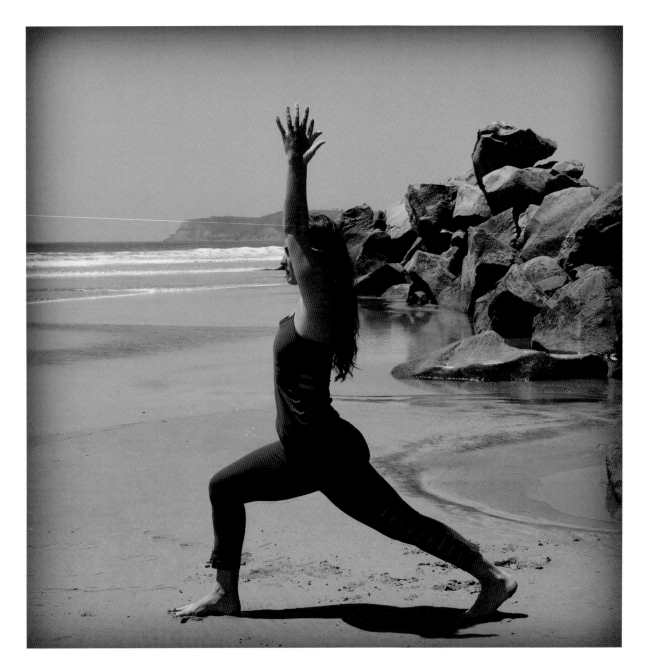

Outfit by Kira Grace – kiragrace.com

"Accept challenges, so that you may feel the exhilaration of victory."
– GEORGE S. PATTON

CRESCENT LUNGE

Begin in Downward-Facing Dog (page 43). With an exhalation, step your right foot forward between your hands.

Bend your front knee to 90 degrees, aligning your knee directly over the heel of your front foot. Your feet should be hip-width apart with both feet facing forward, and your front shin should be perpendicular to the floor.

Shift to the ball of your back foot, lifting your heel and drawing it forward so it aligns over your back toes.

Lift your back leg strongly, drawing your knee and quadriceps up toward the ceiling. Straighten your back leg completely.

With your back leg strong and active, gently draw your left hip forward as you press your right hip back, squaring your hips so they are parallel to the top edge of your mat.

Inhale as you raise your torso to an upright position. Sweep your arms overhead. Draw your tailbone toward the floor. Spin your pinky fingers toward each other, opening your arms so your palms face each other. Make sure your front shin stays vertical. Widen your stance as needed to make sure that your knee does not move forward past your ankle.

Tuck your tailbone under and engage the muscles of your abdomen to help stabilize your core. Extend up through the crown of your head, lengthening your upper body. Draw your shoulder blades firmly into your upper back.

Here is a wholesome way to enjoy a wrap or sandwich. Every ingredient matters and is good for your body. Serve with everything you would serve with mayo. Veggie wraps are my favorite, but tuna salad is a close second.

VEGAN SPICY ALMONDS

Serves 4

3 cups whole unblanched almonds
2½ tablespoons coconut oil
2 teaspoons kosher salt
½ teaspoon freshly ground pepper
½ teaspoon chili powder
½ teaspoon paprika

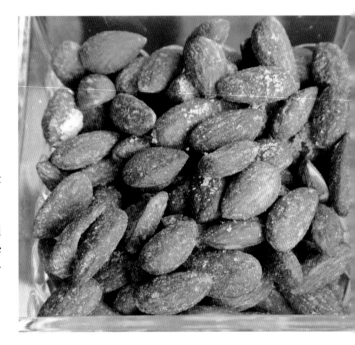

Preheat the oven to 350 degrees F. Line a baking sheet with parchment paper.

In a large bowl, toss together all the ingredients until the nuts are evenly coated. Scatter the nuts onto the baking sheet and bake for 8 minutes. Serve immediately or store in an airtight container.

LOW LUNGE

From Downward-Facing Dog (page 43), exhale and step your right foot forward between your hands, aligning your right knee over your heel. Then, lower your left knee to the floor and, keeping the right knee fixed in place, slide the left back until you feel a comfortable stretch in the left front thigh and groin. Turn the top of your left foot to the floor.

Inhale and lift your torso upright. As you do, sweep your arms out to the sides and up to the sky. Draw your tailbone down toward the floor and lift your pubic bone toward your navel.

Lift your chest and actively reach through your hands.

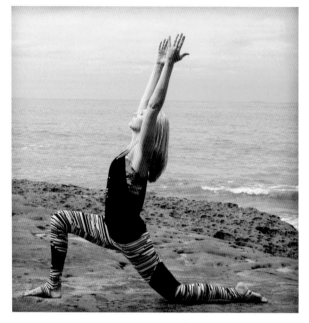

Top by Onzie – onzie.com
Pants by ProperFit – etsy.com/shop/ProperFit

"A chain is as strong as its weakest link."
– UNATTRIBUTED PROVERB

This bread is 100% whole-grain bread. Full of seeds and all things wholesome.

WHOLE-GRAIN BREAD

Makes 1 loaf

1½ cups lukewarm water
2 tablespoons butter or vegetable oil
1½ teaspoons salt
2 tablespoons pure cane sugar
½ cup nonfat dry milk
3 cups organic, stone-ground whole-wheat flour
¼ cup chia seeds
¼ cup old fashioned oats
¼ cup flax seeds
¼ cup sesame seeds
1 tablespoon instant yeast
2 tablespoons vital wheat gluten

Combine all of the ingredients, mix, and knead—by hand, mixer, or bread machine—until you've made a smooth dough. Place it in a lightly greased bowl, cover the bowl, and allow it to rise for 60 to 90 minutes until it's expanded a bit. It won't have doubled in size, but should feel puffy when you squeeze it.

Lightly grease a 9 × 5–inch loaf pan. Gently shape the dough into a smooth log.

Place it in the pan smooth side up, cover the pan, and allow the loaf to rise for about 30 to 45 minutes. Towards the end of the rising time, preheat the oven to 375 degrees F.

Bake the bread for 35 to 40 minutes. Remove it from the oven, and turn it out of the pan onto a rack. Allow the bread to cool completely before slicing. Slice and store in an airtight container in the fridge. Don't forget to eat a fresh piece first!

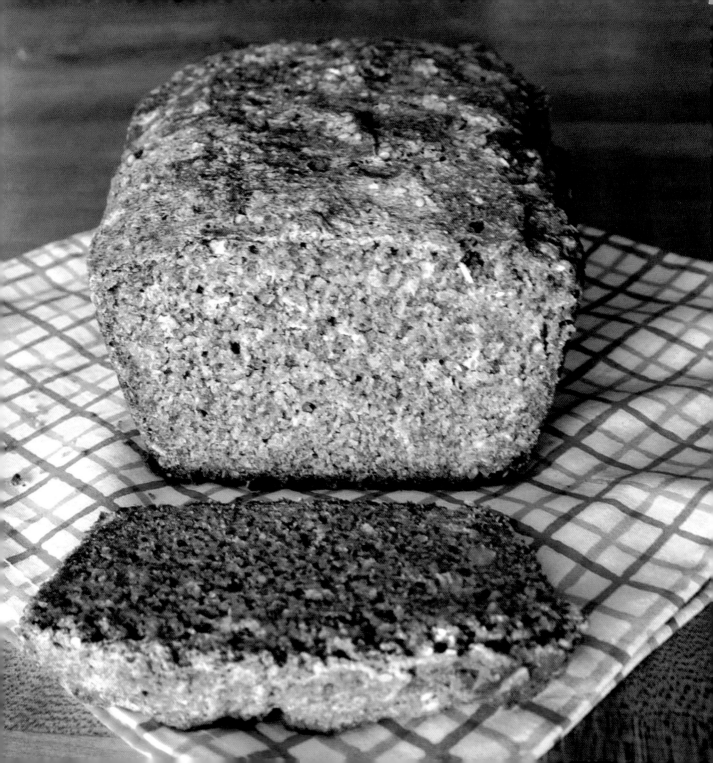

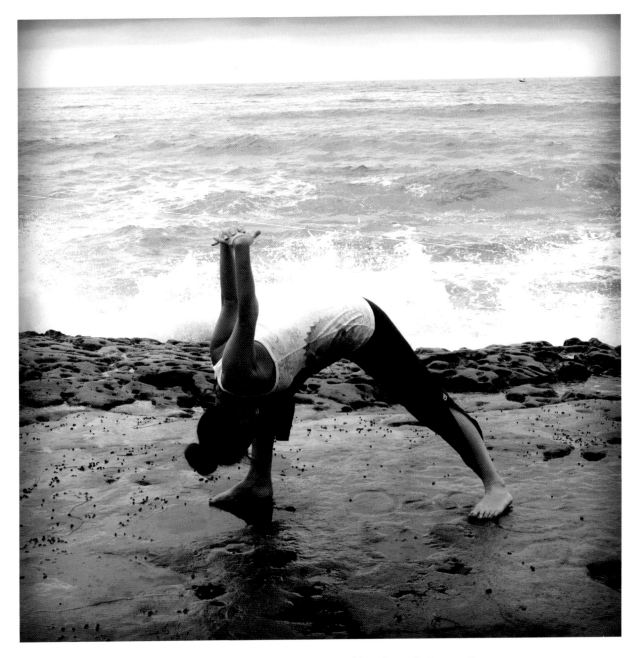

Top by Cocoon by Susanne B – etsy.com/shop/CocoonBySuzanneB
Pants by Be Present – bepresent.com

HUMBLE WARRIOR

Begin in Mountain Pose (page 17). Step feet apart, taking a wide stance. Pivot left foot out about 45 degrees.

Turn torso right, square hips, bend right knee, and pivot right foot out so it points ahead in alignment with knee. Bend knee forward until thigh is parallel to floor. Draw shoulder blades together and down.

Reach arms above head, palms facing each other, lengthening spine. Gently arch back while gazing upward. To come out, lower hands while straightening front leg and push back into Mountain Pose. Repeat on left side.

Release the arms and bring them behind your back, interlacing the fingers in preparation for Humble Warrior. Reach the interlaced finger down your back to open your chest before forward-bending your upper body inside your right knee. The arms go up toward the sky and your head reaches for the floor. Try to keep your front knee deep and the hips squared to the front; avoid resting your weight on the front knee.

"To keep our faces toward change, and behave like free spirits in the presence of fate, is strength undefeatable."
– HELEN KELLER

Watch others stuff their faces with potato chips while your zucchini chips work on your figure.

BAKED ZUCCHINI CHIPS

Serves 1

1 zucchini
sea salt

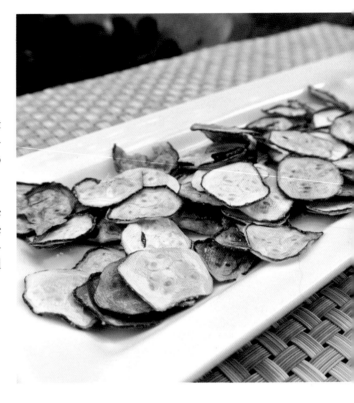

Preheat oven to 225 degrees F. Line a baking sheet with parchment paper and set aside. Using your mandoline slicer on the thinnest setting, slice zucchini into thin medallions.

Lay out slices on prepared baking sheet and sprinkle lightly with sea salt. Place in preheated oven and bake for one hour. Rotate baking sheet and bake an additional 20 minutes, until chips are browned and crisped to your liking. Serve right away!

WARRIOR 1

Begin in Mountain Pose (page 17). Step feet apart, taking a wide stance. Pivot left foot out about 45 degrees.

Turn torso right, square hips, bend right knee, and pivot right foot out so it points ahead in alignment with knee. Bend knee forward until thigh is parallel to floor. Draw shoulder blades together and down.

Reach arms above head, palms facing each other, and lengthen your spine. Gently arch your back while gazing upward. To come out, lower hands while straightening front leg and push back into Mountain Pose. Repeat on left side.

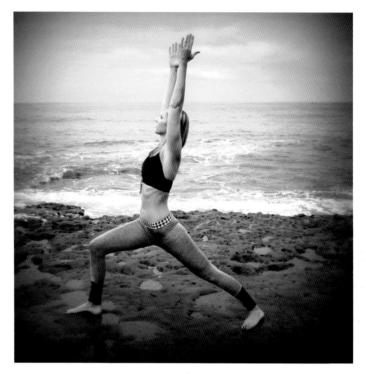

Outfit by ProperFit – etsy.com/shop/ProperFit

"How can something bother you if you won't let it?"
– TERRI GUILLEMETS

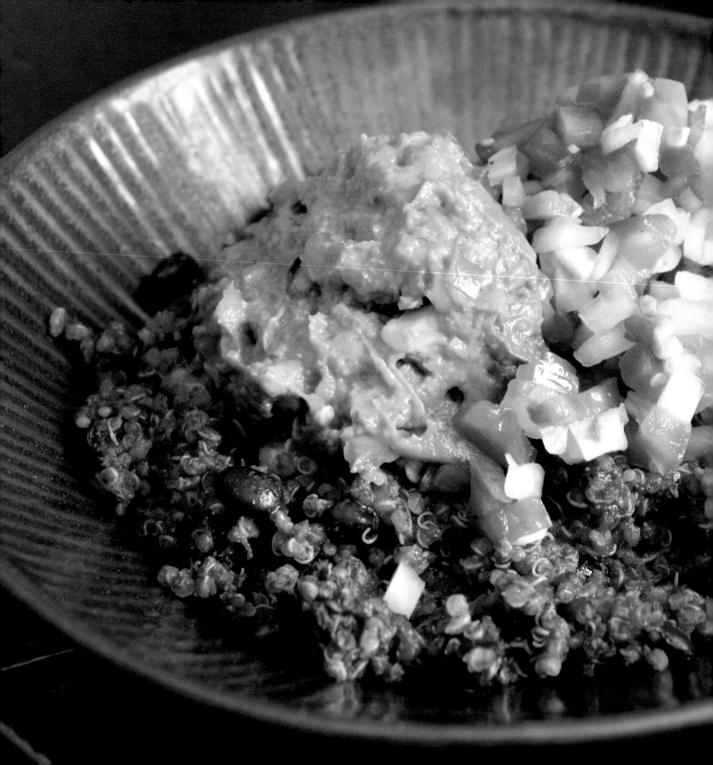

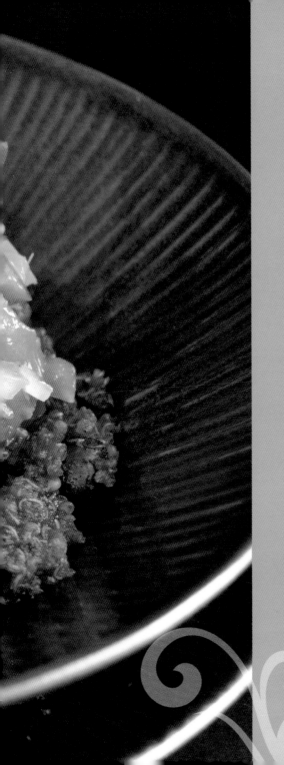

FEED THE MACHINE

Another mistake so many people make when starting their healthy eating is not eating enough. They get caught up on fats rather than calories. It is so important to have a good amount of healthy fat in our diets. Nuts, avocados, and coconut oil are my top 3 sources for healthy fats. Try to stop looking at fat content and look at the ingredients. Everything you put in your body should have a purpose. These recipes have been approved by the pickiest eaters and they are designed to feed the machine.

This bowl is packed full of all the nutrients you need to start your day off right.

AÇAÍ BOWL

Serves 2

2 tablespoons coconut oil
¼ cup unsweetened coconut flakes
¼ cup pumpkin seeds
¼ cup cashew meal
¼ cup almond meal
¼ cup oats
¼ cup raw honey
1 sweet ripe banana
½ cup açaí powder
½ cup plain Greek yogurt
½ cup almond milk
fresh berries and banana slices for topping
optional mint for garnish

Heat the coconut oil in a pan on medium-high heat. Toss the coconut, oats, and all the nuts in the pan and coat in the oil. Stir them continuously. Watch them very closely, as they can burn quickly. You want the coconut to brown. Once the nuts are toasted, remove from heat, stir in the honey, and then let them cool.

Put the banana in the blender with the açaí powder, yogurt, and almond milk. Start the blender on low then ramp it up to max. Blend for 1 to 2 minutes. Pour equal parts berry blend and nut mixture in bowl.

Top with banana slices, berries, and optional mint for garnish!

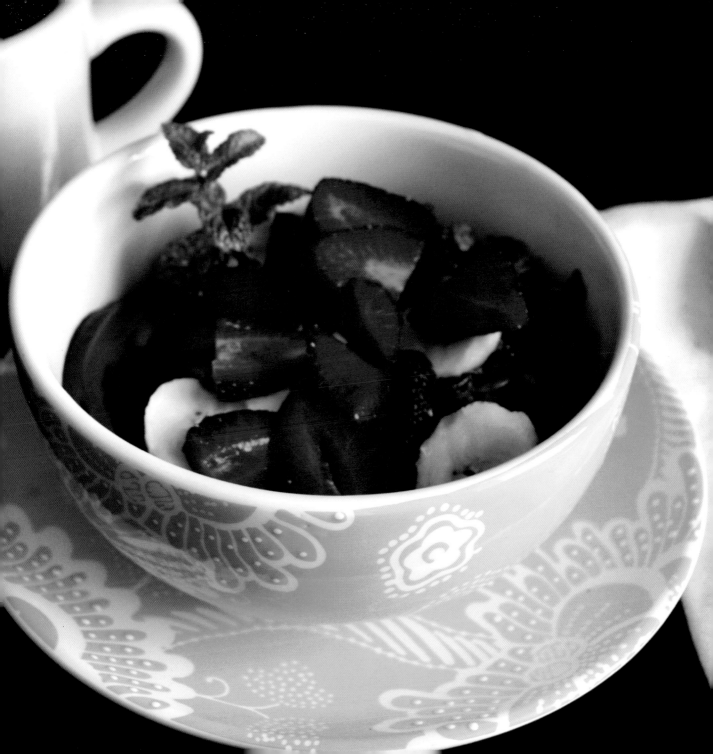

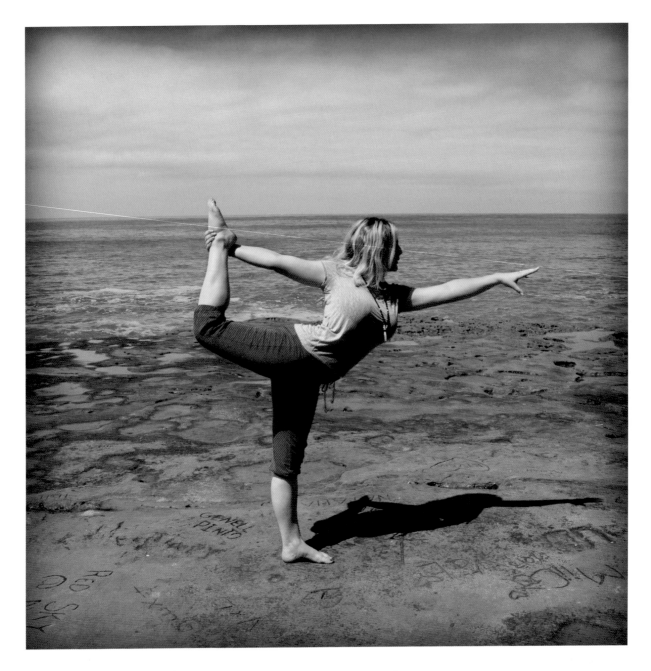

Outfit by Green Apple Active – greenappleactive.com

DANCER POSE

Begin standing in Mountain Pose (page 17) with your feet together and your arms at your sides. Shift your weight onto your left foot.

Bend your right knee and bring your right heel toward your right buttock. Reach your right hand down and clasp your right foot's inner ankle. You can also loop a strap around the top of your right foot, and then hold onto the strap with your right hand. Draw your knees together.

Reach your left arm out in front of you, pointing your fingertips forward with your palm facing down.

Fix your gaze softly at an unmoving spot in front of you. Make sure your left kneecap and toes continue to point directly forward.

When you feel steady and comfortable, begin to press your right foot away from your body as you simultaneously lean your torso slightly forward. Keep your chest lifting and continue reaching your left hand's fingertips up toward the ceiling.

Raise your right foot as high as you can. Bring your left thigh parallel to the floor, or higher if possible. At the same time, press your tailbone toward the floor to avoid compressing your lower back. Do not let your right knee splay open to the side.

"You may not control all the events that happen to you, but you can decide not to be reduced by them."
– MAYA ANGELOU

These are great served by themselves, or I serve mine over super greens and homemade ranch.

ALMOND-CRUSTED CHICKEN STRIPS

Serves 4

1 cup raw almonds
2 teaspoons paprika
¼ cup Parmesan cheese
1 teaspoon Italian seasoning
1 teaspoon salt
½ teaspoon pepper
1 pound boneless, skinless chicken breast
1 egg
olive oil
optional:
greens
ranch

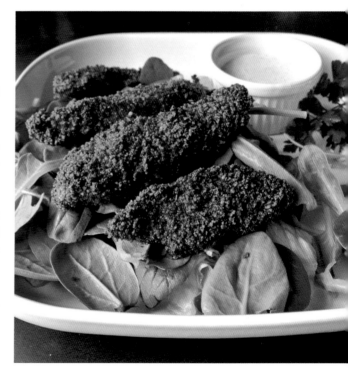

Preheat oven to 425 degrees F. Grind up your almonds in a food processor until they resemble bread crumbs.

Mix together the ground almonds, paprika, Parmesan, Italian seasoning, salt, and pepper into a shallow dish and set aside.

Rinse chicken and pat dry with paper towels, then cut into even-sized long portions. Whisk your egg. Coat each piece of chicken with egg, then dip evenly into the almond mixture.

Place each chicken strip on a lined baking sheet and drizzle or spray lightly with olive oil. Bake for 20–22 minutes, until golden brown and crisp on the outside.

"If you can find a path with no obstacles, it probably doesn't lead anywhere."
— ATTRIBUTED TO FRANK A. CLARK

PYRAMID POSE

Stand in Mountain Pose (page 17) at the back of your mat. Step your right foot forward 3 feet and place your hands on your hips. Your right foot should face forward. Turn your left foot out 45 degrees to the right for stability. Align the right heel with the left heel.

Square hips with the front of the mat. Reach upward and lengthen the spine on an inhale. Exhale and come forward, bending at the hip. Bring your hands to floor, or for a deeper stretch that helps keep the shoulders back, you can grab either elbow behind your back as shown in the picture.

Lengthen the spine on each inhale. On each exhale, bend forward a little deeper. Come up and repeat on the left side.

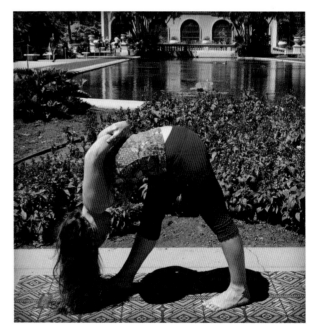

Outfit by Hotdrop – hotdropapparel.com

Try making this crispy crust with ground-up almonds. Shock everyone with this packed-with-protein pizza. You can't taste the nuts!

ALMOND CRUST PIZZA

Makes 1 (12-inch) pizza crust
2 cups almond meal
2 eggs
3 tablespoons olive oil
¼ teaspoon baking soda
1 teaspoon garlic powder
1 tablespoon Italian seasoning

TOPPINGS:
1 cup marinara sauce
1 cup shredded mozzarella
fresh veggies of your choice
toppings of your choice

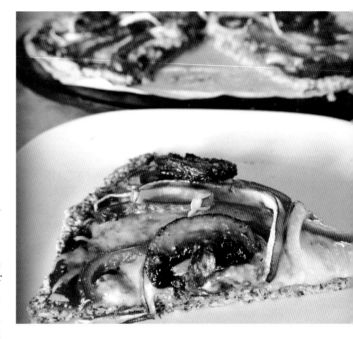

Preheat your oven to 350 degrees F. Using a spoon, mix all crust ingredients together until it becomes very thick. Using your hands, form the dough into a ball.

Lightly grease a pizza pan or a baking stone with olive oil, or cover with parchment paper. Place the ball of dough in the center of your cookie sheet or pizza pan and, using your hands, push and pat the dough down into the shape of a circle. Pressing until the dough is flat and 12 inches across. Bake the crust in your pre-heated oven for 20 minutes.

While your crust is cooking, prepare your toppings. After the crust is done, remove from the oven and evenly spread the marinara sauce over the crust.

Finish topping the pizza with cheese and the rest of your favorite toppings. I went for a vegetarian pizza with red onion, peppers, and mushrooms. But you can put whatever you choose on. Bake again for an additional 25 minutes. Slice and serve.

GODDESS POSE

Begin in Mountain Pose (page 17). Turn to the right and step your feet wide apart. Turn your toes out slightly so that they point to the corners of your mat.

Exhale, bend your knees directly over your toes, and lower your hips into a squat. Work toward bringing your thighs as parallel to the floor as you can.

Extend your arms out to the sides at shoulder-height with your palms facing down. Then, spiral your thumbs up toward the ceiling so that your palms face forward. Bend your elbows and point your fingertips toward the ceiling; your upper arms and forearms should be at a 90-degree angle.

Tuck your tailbone in slightly and press your hips forward as you draw your thighs back. Keep your knees in line with your toes.

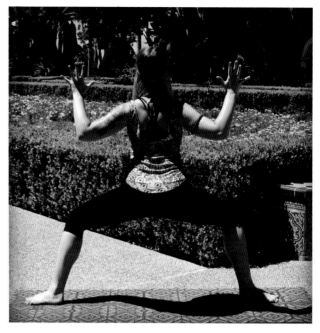

Outfit by Onzie – onzie.com
Mat by Optimistic Elephant – etsy.com/shop/OptimisticElephant

"What you're supposed to do when you don't like a thing is change it. If you can't change it, change the way you think about it."
– MAYA ANGELOU

One easy way to cut down on calories is to use lettuce as your wrap, rather than carb-loaded options. When the filling is full of flavor, you won't miss it!

ASIAN LETTUCE CUPS

Serves 4

1 tablespoon sesame oil
1 pound chicken breasts, chopped
1 clove garlic, minced
⅛ teaspoon ground ginger
⅔ cup thinly sliced green onions
1 (8-ounce) can sliced water chestnuts, drained and coarsely chopped
3 tablespoons Healthy Hoisin Sauce (page 174)
2 tablespoons soy sauce (or Bragg's amino acids)
1 tablespoon rice vinegar
2 teaspoons roasted red chili paste
12 butter lettuce leaves

Heat 1 tablespoon of oil in a large nonstick skillet over medium-high heat. Add chicken, garlic, and ginger to the pan and cook for about 6 minutes or until chicken is cooked through.

Combine chicken mixture, onions, and chopped water chestnuts in a large bowl, stirring well, and set aside.

In a small bowl, whisk together hoisin, soy sauce, rice vinegar, and roasted red chili paste and drizzle over the cooked chicken mixture. Toss to coat completely. Add about ¼ cup chicken mixture to each lettuce leaf, serve, and enjoy!

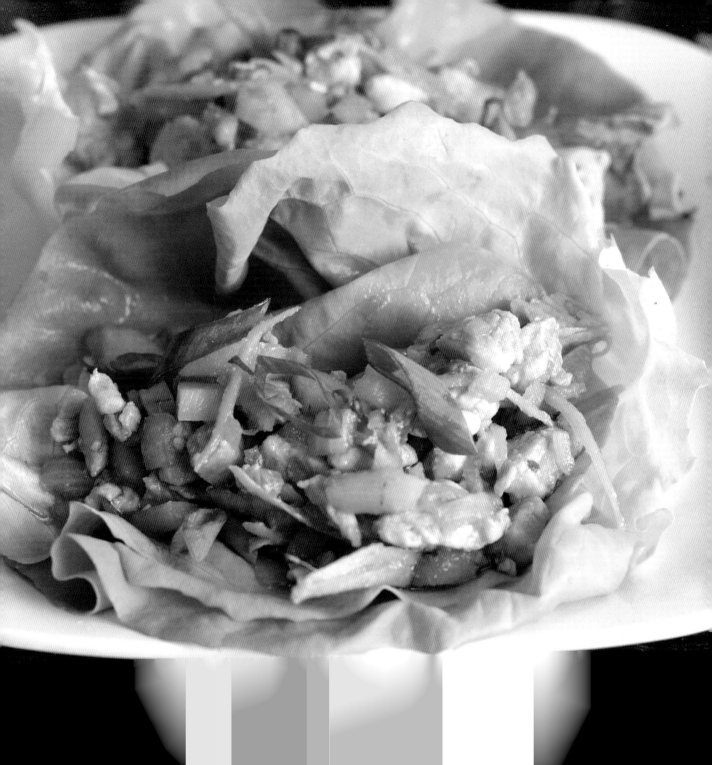

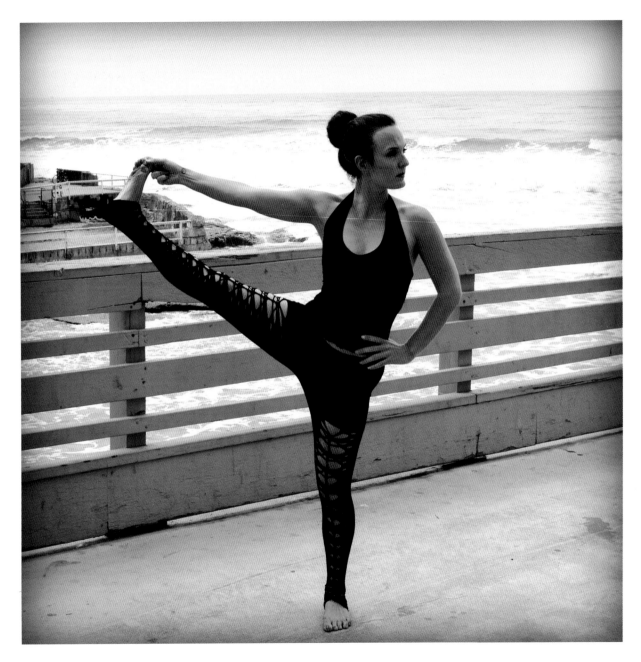

Top by Shantari – etsy.com/shop/SHANTARI
Leggings by 4TheWild – etsy.com/shop/4TheWild

> "It's not whether you get knocked down, it's whether you get up."
> **– VINCE LOMBARDI**

STANDING HAND-TO-BIG-TOE POSE

Begin in Mountain Pose (page 17). Shift your weight to your left foot. Very slowly, draw your right knee up toward your chest. Bring your right arm to the inside of your right thigh. Then loop your index and middle fingers around your right foot's big toe. Place your left hand on your left hip.

Straighten your spine. Strongly engage your abdominal muscles and the muscles of your left leg. Straighten your left leg, but do not lock your knee.

On an exhalation, extend your right leg forward, grabbing on to your big toe with your peace fingers. Straighten your right leg as much as possible.

Keep both hips squared forward and keep your spine straight. If you are stable and strong here, you can widen your leg out to the side and stand tall.

This meal is perfect for nights you need to get dinner on in less than 20 minutes. So tasty it will impress everyone at the table.

BLACKENED SALMON

Serves 4

1 teaspoon garlic salt
1 teaspoon paprika
1 teaspoon onion powder
1 teaspoon oregano
1 teaspoon black pepper
½ teaspoon cayenne pepper
½ teaspoon thyme
2 pounds salmon, cut into 8-ounce filets
2 tablespoons olive oil

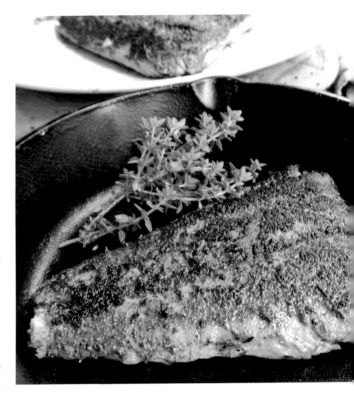

Combine garlic salt, paprika, onion powder, oregano, black pepper, cayenne pepper, and thyme. Mix it together and rub mixture on both sides of fish.

Heat a large cast-iron skillet over medium-high heat. Add olive oil and seasoned fish.

Cook 5 to 8 minutes on each side, or until fish flakes easily with a fork. Serve over your favorite greens, rice, or quinoa.

GARLAND POSE

Squat with your feet as close together as possible while keeping your heels on the floor.

Separate your thighs slightly wider than your torso. Exhaling, lean your torso forward and fit it snugly between your thighs.

Press your elbows against your inner knees, bringing your palms together, and resist the knees into the elbows. This will help lengthen your front torso.

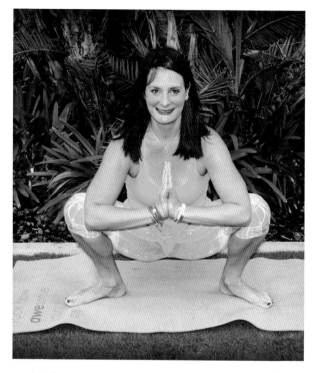

Top by Green Apple Activewear – greenappleactive.com
Capri Leggings by Luna Jai – lunajai.com
Necklace by Bliss in Art – etsy.com/shop/BlissInArt
Mat by AffirMats – affirmats.com/

"The only thing that overcomes hard luck is hard work."
– HARRY GOLDEN

The creamy avocado replaces cheese in this healthy vegan pasta recipe. For those not wanting to be vegan, just add cooked chicken for extra protein.

CAPRESE PASTA

Serves 2

1 box quinoa fettuccine
2 tomatoes, cubed
1 avocado, peeled, pit removed, and cubed
1 cup chopped, fresh basil leaves
¼ cup balsamic vinegar
1 teaspoon garlic salt

Cook your quinoa pasta according to package directions. While pasta is cooking, prepare your vegetables.

Drain pasta and pour into a large bowl. Top with veggies, balsamic vinegar, and garlic salt. Toss to coat. (If you want more protein, this is where you add cooked chicken.) Serve!

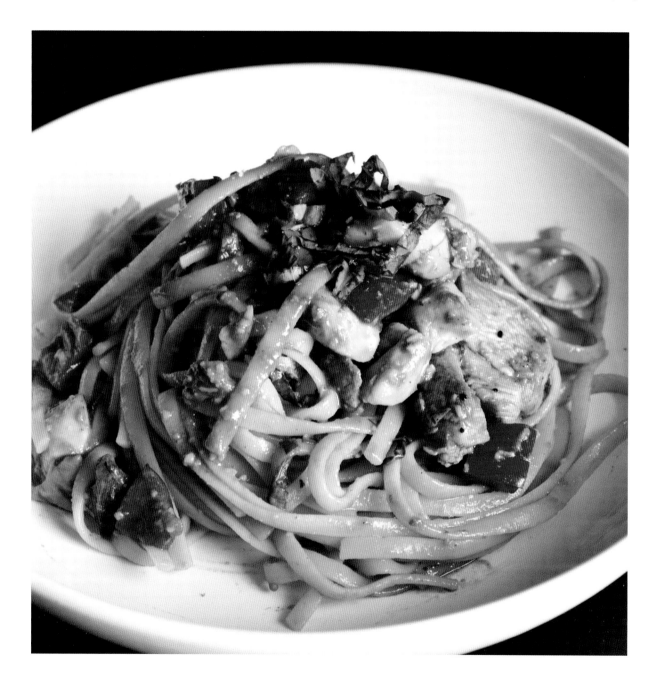

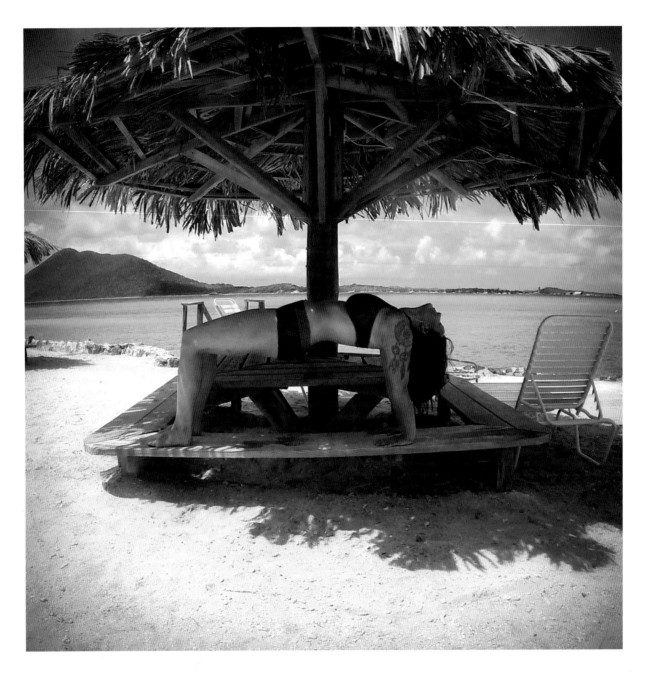

Suit by Dragonfly – dragonfly-yogawear.com

REVERSE TABLETOP

Begin by sitting on the floor with your legs extended in front of you and your arms resting at your sides in a seated Staff Pose (page 137). Bend your knees and place your feet flat on the floor.

Place your hands several inches behind your hips, shoulder-width apart. Press your palms flat, and turn your fingertips inward toward your toes.

Inhaling, press firmly into your hands and feet. Straighten your elbows and lift your hips up toward the sky. Draw your shoulder blades firmly into your back and lift your chest. Try to bring your chest, torso, and knees into one straight line, parallel to the floor.

Keep your legs active and firm, but do not squeeze your buttocks. Press down through all ten toes.

Gently drop your head back so the crown of your head faces the floor. Breathe.

"We must embrace pain and burn it as fuel for our journey."
– KENJI MIYAZAWA

This is my go-to comfort food. It makes me feel like I am getting away with something, when in reality it is packed with nutrients and protein. Ditch the rice. Quinoa is where it is at!

VEGETARIAN CHICKEN-FRIED QUINOA

Serves 4

3 teaspoons canola oil
1 tablespoon minced garlic
¾ teaspoon salt
¼ teaspoon black pepper
½ cup chopped onion
2 tablespoons chopped green onion (optional more for garnish)
½ cup chopped carrots
2 eggs, beaten
4 cups Perfectly Cooked Quinoa (page 60)
¼ cup Bragg's amino acids or gluten-free soy sauce
salt and pepper to taste

Heat a nonstick skillet over medium heat. Add 1 teaspoon of oil, garlic, salt, and pepper. Add the remaining 2 tablespoons of oil to the pan and raise the heat to medium-high. Sauté the onion, green onion, and carrots until tender, 2–3 minutes.

Move cooked veggies to the side of the pan. Add the beaten eggs to the skillet and scramble the eggs until they're firm.

Mix together the quinoa, scrambled eggs, and veggies, stirring well. Add the Bragg's amino acids or gluten-free soy sauce to the mixture. Let cook for a few minutes, then flip over. Cook for another few minutes until a little crispy. Stir together. Top with optional green onions for garnish and serve!

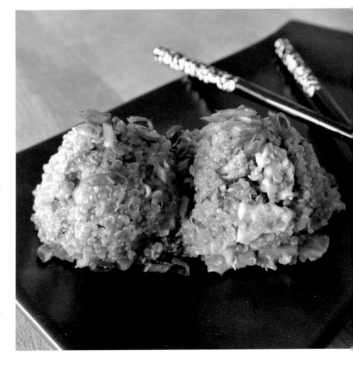

> "When life gives you a hundred reasons to cry, show life that you have
> a thousand reasons to smile."
> **– UNKNOWN**

TIGER POSE

Begin in Tabletop Pose (see page 111). Exhale and reach your right foot up towards the ceiling with the knee bent and the spine gently arching.

Staring at a point straight ahead, shift your weight into your right hand and carefully reach the left hand to hold on to the inside of the right ankle.

With both arms straight, gently kick the right foot into the left arm to lift the leg higher. Repeat on the other side.

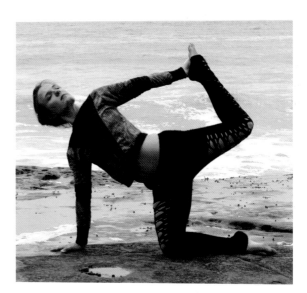

Top by ProperFit – etsy.com/shop/ProperFit
Leggings by 4theWild – etsy.com/shop/4theWild

I love this dish It is tangy and spicy and makes my taste buds dance. Not only that, but it is healthy—full of God-given nutrients, protein, and healthy fat.

CITRUS CHICKEN WITH AVOCADO BLACK BEAN SALAD

Serves 4

FOR CHICKEN:
3 oranges, juiced
3 limes, juiced
½ bunch of cilantro, chopped
1 jalapeño, sliced
1 teaspoon of kosher salt
4 chicken breasts or 12 tenders
¼ cup olive oil
2 cloves of garlic
4 slices of jack or pepper jack cheese

FOR AVOCADO BLACK BEAN SALAD:
3 avocados, diced
1 cup of cherry tomatoes, diced
½ red onion, diced
1 can of black beans, drained and rinsed
1 jalapeño, diced
2 limes
1 teaspoon cumin
salt and pepper to taste

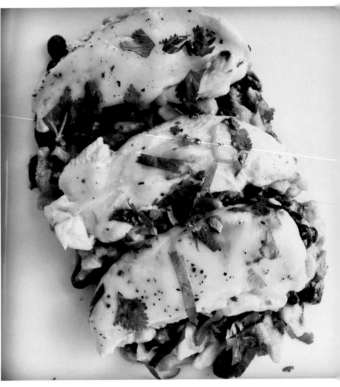

In a large ziplock bag or bowl, combine orange juice, lime juice, cilantro, jalapeño, and salt and mix well. Add chicken breasts and marinate for at least 2 hours.

To make the Avocado Black Bean Salad, combine avocados, cherry tomatoes, red onion, black beans, jalapeño, juice of 1½ limes, and cumin to a bowl and mix to combine. Don't overmix; you want the avocado to remain chunky. Salt and pepper to taste.

Preheat oven to broil. Combine olive oil and minced garlic cloves in a small bowl and set aside. Mix olive oil and garlic together and then brush onto the chicken breasts. Broil on high for 5 minutes, then add cheese slices to the top of the chicken and broil for another minute to melt cheese.

Serve Citrus Chicken over Avocado Black Bean Salad and garnish with cilantro.

CAT/COW POSE

Begin in Tabletop Pose (see page 111) with wrists under shoulders and knees under hips, with the back flat in neutral spine and abs engaged.

Deeply inhale. Exhale into Cat Pose and round spine towards ceiling, pulling navel in towards spine and engaging the abs. Tuck chin to chest, allowing neck to release.

Inhale to Cow Pose, arch back, and let belly relax and loosen. Lift head and tailbone up towards ceiling. Continue flowing back and forth from Cat to Cow, inhaling for Cow Pose and exhale on Cat Pose. Repeat for 5–10 rounds or until your spine is warmed up.

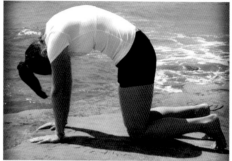
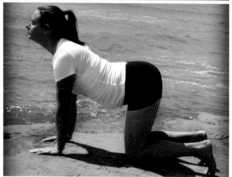

Outfit by Green Apple Activewear – greenappleactive.com

The addition of almonds to this classic vegetarian dish adds more protein, and the desired outside crunch is nicely balanced by the soft delicate inside—making meat lovers love it!

ALMOND FALAFEL WRAP

Serves 4

2 cups garbanzo beans or chickpeas
¼ cup fresh mint, chopped
¼ cup green onions sliced.
¼ cup shredded carrots
¼ cup fresh parsley
2 cloves garlic
2 tablespoons olive oil
1 tablespoon fresh lemon juice
1 tablespoon sriracha
1 teaspoon cumin
1 teaspoon coriander
½ teaspoon salt
1½ tablespoons chickpea flour
1 cup almond meal
1 teaspoon garlic salt
¼ cup grapeseed oil
your favorite wrap, pita bread, or tortilla
lettuce
Greek Drizzle Sauce (page 170)

Preheat your oven to 400 degrees F. Place the chickpeas in a food processor and process until they resemble the consistency of rough-cut bread crumbs. Stir in everything from the fresh mint through the chickpea flour.

Create golf ball–sized balls out of the dough created. Combine the almond meal and garlic salt in a shallow dish. Roll the balls you created in the almond meal mixture.

In a skillet, heat up the grapeseed oil. Brown the outside of your falafel balls in the hot oil and then place in a shallow baking dish. Bake your falafels for 15–20 minutes.

To assemble, place your wrap on the table and top with the desired amount of Greek Drizzle Sauce. I usually use 2 tablespoons. Add lettuce and your falafel balls. Wrap up, cut in half, and serve.

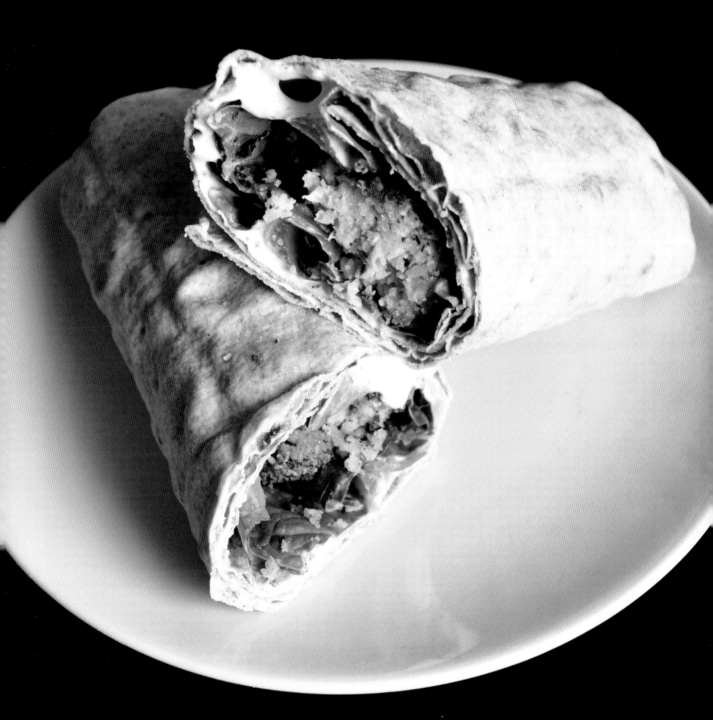

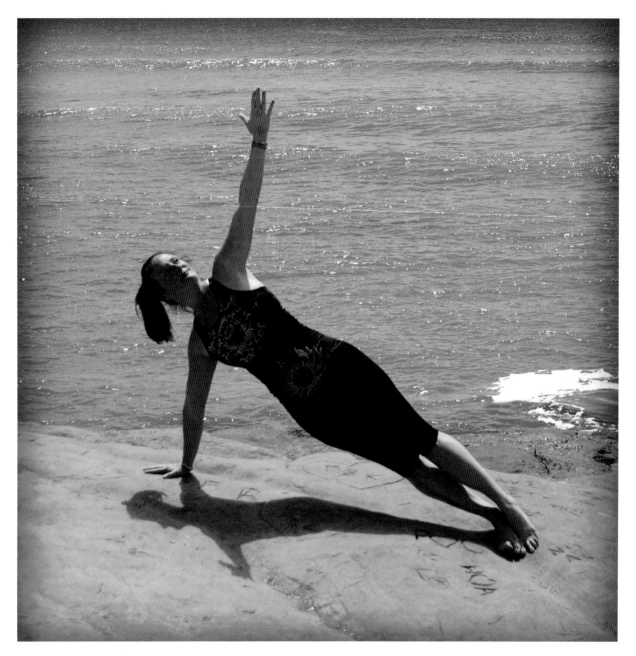

Top by YMX by Yellowman – ymxbyellowman.com
Pants by Green Apple Active – greenappleactive.com

"How you think about a problem is more important than the problem itself. So always think positively."
– **NORMAN VINCENT PEALE**

SIDE PLANK

Begin in Downward-Facing Dog (page 43). Lower your hips and shift your weight forward to come into Plank Pose (page 33); this resembles the top of a push-up. Keep your palms flat and body extended with your legs reaching through your heels.

Step your feet together and press your weight down through your right hand and forearm. Then, roll your body to the right, balancing on the outer edge of your right foot. Stack your left foot on top of your right foot and keep your legs straight.

Extend your left arm to the sky, reaching through your fingertips as you lift your hips and firm the triceps of both arms. Feel the muscles across your shoulder blades flex.

Firm your thighs, and press through your heels into the floor. Bring your body into one straight line. Gaze at your top thumb. Press down through your bottom index finger.

This is a dish that will make everyone think you spent hours in the kitchen, but in reality it takes less than 10 minutes to prepare.

GLAZED SCALLOP CUCUMBER SALAD

Serves 1

1 cucumber
1 tablespoon sesame oil
6 jumbo sea scallops
salt and pepper to taste
2 teaspoons canola oil
1 tablespoon prepared hoisin sauce

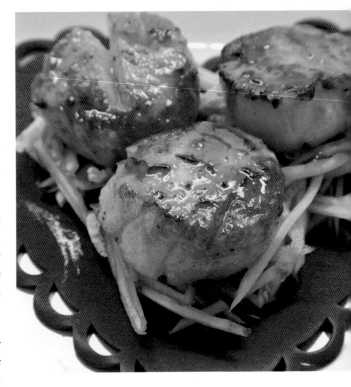

Peel and julienne cut a cucumber. This is done easily with a mandoline. Toss cut cucumber with sesame oil and place on a plate.

Make sure scallops are completely clean and that the side muscle is not still attached. If it is, pull it off and discard. Bring the scallops to room temperature by drying them with a paper towel and setting them aside for about 30 minutes. Season the scallops with salt and pepper.

Heat heavy-bottomed sauté or frying pan over medium-high heat. Once pan is hot, add oil. Place scallops in pan flat-side down. Don't crowd them. Leave scallops alone and don't move them for 2–3 minutes. Turn scallops over, turn heat down, and drizzle with hoisin sauce. Cook 1 more minute. Serve immediately over prepared cucumber.

UPWARD PLANK POSE

Begin in Staff Pose (page 137) with your hands several inches behind your hips and your fingers pointing forward. Bend your knees and place your feet on the floor, big toes turned inward, heels at least a foot away from your buttocks.

Exhale, press your inner feet and hands down against the floor, and lift your hips until you come into a Reverse Tabletop position (page 111), torso and thighs parallel to the floor, shins and arms perpendicular.

Without losing the height of your hips, straighten your legs one at a time. Lift your hips even higher without hardening your buttocks. Press your shoulder blades against your back torso to support the lift of your chest.

Without compressing the back of your neck, slowly drop your head back.

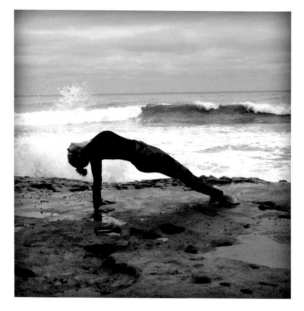

Outfit by ProperFit – etsy.com/shop/ProperFit

"If you cannot get rid of the family skeleton, you may as well make it dance."
– GEORGE BERNARD SHAW

This dish is so amazing, everyone will think you are a gourmet chef. Don't be overwhelmed; it is easy to make if you follow the steps!

KALE, POTATO, AND SMOKED GOUDA QUICHE

CRUST:
1½ tablespoons olive oil
2 packed cups shredded russet potatoes
1 small onion, shredded
¼ teaspoon salt

FILLING:
1 tablespoon olive oil
2 cups kale, removed from stem, chopped,
    and packed
1 sweet onion
⅔ cup chopped chives
3 eggs
½ cup plain Greek yogurt
⅔ cup smoked Gouda cheese, grated and packed
¼ teaspoon salt
¼ teaspoon pepper

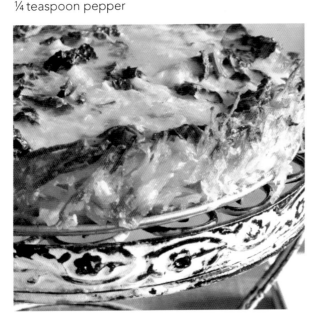

Preheat oven to 425 degrees F. Grease a 9-inch pie dish or a springform pan with olive oil. Set aside.

Place the shredded potatoes and onion in a strainer and drain very well. I recommend doing this the night before. It takes several hours for the potatoes to dry. Soggy taters = soggy crust. The shreds will turn brown upon oxidation, but they turn brown when you cook them anyway. This in no way will affect the taste or texture of the potatoes. I put mine in a strainer, cover it with plastic wrap, and put over a bowl in the fridge overnight. After draining, use your hands to gently squeeze out any remaining water. In a large bowl, using your hands, mix the shreds with the salt and oil. Press into the pan firmly. Bake the crust for 30 minutes. Remove from heat and set aside.

Reduce oven heat to 350 degrees and prepare your filling. In a skillet, heat 1 tablespoon olive oil over medium-high heat. Add in kale and cook for 1 minute, stirring and tossing frequently. Add in sweet onion and chives and cook, stirring and tossing frequently, for another 2 minutes. Turn off heat and set skillet aside.

In a bowl, whisk together eggs, Greek yogurt, smoked Gouda, salt, and pepper.

Add in sautéed kale, sweet onion, and chives. Whisk everything together. Pour into baked hash brown pie crust. Bake for 35–40 minutes, or until egg mixture is set. Allow to cool at least 10 minutes before slicing.

WILD THING

From Downward-Facing Dog (page 43), come into a Side Plank (page 119) on your right side. Step your left foot behind you, keep your right leg straight, and push your hips up away from the floor.

Scoop your tailbone and use your legs to keep lifting your hips. Curl your head back, lift the left side of your body, and keep your left upper arm moving toward your shoulder socket.

Extend your left arm over your head and curve into a back bend. When you are done being wild, release, step back to Downward-Facing Dog, and switch sides.

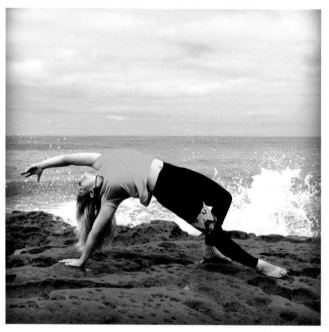

Top by Green Apple Activewear – greenappleactive.com
Pants by Proper Fit – etsy.com/shop/properfit

"Change the way you look at things, and the things you look at change."
– WAYNE DYER

The crispy quinoa patties go so nicely with the Greek yogurt and veggies.

MEDITERRANEAN QUINOA WRAPS

Serves 4

2 cups Perfectly Cooked Quinoa (page 60)
½ teaspoon salt
¾ cup shredded cheddar cheese
½ cup ricotta cheese
1 medium carrot, finely grated
3 eggs
3 tablespoons sorghum flour
2 green onions, sliced thin on the bias
½ teaspoon Splenda, sugar, or stevia
¼ teaspoon black pepper
¼ teaspoon ground cumin
⅛ teaspoon garlic powder
olive oil for frying
flax wrap, whole wheat tortilla, or lavash bread
sliced cucumber
sliced tomato
sliced red pepper
Greek Drizzle Sauce (page 170)

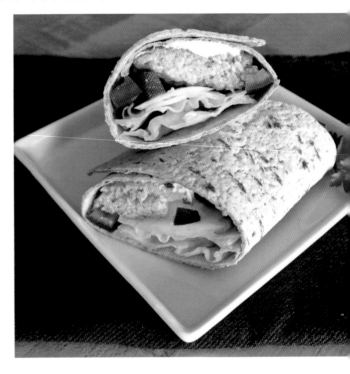

In a large bowl combine the cooked quinoa, salt, cheddar cheese, ricotta cheese, carrot, eggs, sorghum flour, green onions, Splenda, pepper, cumin, and garlic powder. Mix well and then let chill in the fridge for 1 hour to let it set.

Heat a frying pan or griddle and a couple teaspoons of olive oil over medium-low heat. Mixture will be slightly sticky, so use a ¼-cup measuring cup to drop mixture into pan and lightly flatten to ½-inch thick. I make mine long and oval-shaped to fit in a wrap.

Fry until golden-brown, about 4 minutes on each side. You can store them in between parchment paper in an airtight container until you are ready to serve.

Using a flax wrap, whole wheat tortilla, or lavash bread, add cucumber, tomato, and red pepper. I added chives, too, for extra flavor. Add quinoa patties. Top with Greek Drizzle Sauce. Wrap to close and serve!

"In one minute you can change your attitude, and in that minute you can change your entire day."
– SPENCER JOHNSON

LOCUST POSE

Lie on your belly with your arms along the sides of your torso, palms up, forehead resting on the floor. Turn your big toes toward each other to inwardly rotate your thighs.

Exhale and lift your head, upper torso, arms, and legs away from the floor. You will be resting on your lower ribs, belly, and front pelvis. Firm your buttocks and reach strongly through your legs, first through the heels to lengthen the back legs, then through the bases of the big toes. Keep the big toes turned toward each other.

Raise your arms parallel to the floor and stretch back actively through your fingertips. Imagine there is a weight pressing down on the backs of the upper arms, and push up toward the ceiling against this resistance.

Gaze forward or slightly upward, being careful not to jut your chin forward and crunch the back of your neck. Keep the base of the skull lifted and the back of the neck long.

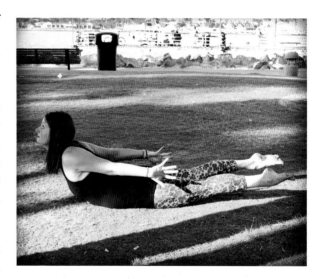

Top by Be Present – bepresent.com
Pants by Liza Jane Apparel – etsy.com/shop/lizajanehandmade

What I love so much about these omelettes is that you can cater them to individual tastes. If someone likes onions, add them. If they don't, leave them out. Throw whatever veggies you like in them!

OVEN-BAKED OMELETTES

Serves 4

8 eggs
1 cup milk
½ teaspoon salt
1 onion, diced
1 red pepper, seeded and diced
4 green onions, sliced
1 cup shredded jack cheese, divided
¼ teaspoon pepper

In a large bowl, beat eggs. Add the milk, salt, onion, and red pepper.

Pour mixture into 4 individual baking dishes or ramekins. Top with sliced green onions.

Bake, uncovered, at 350 degrees F for 30 minutes. Take out and sprinkle with cheese and pepper. Bake another 10 minutes. Serve warm.

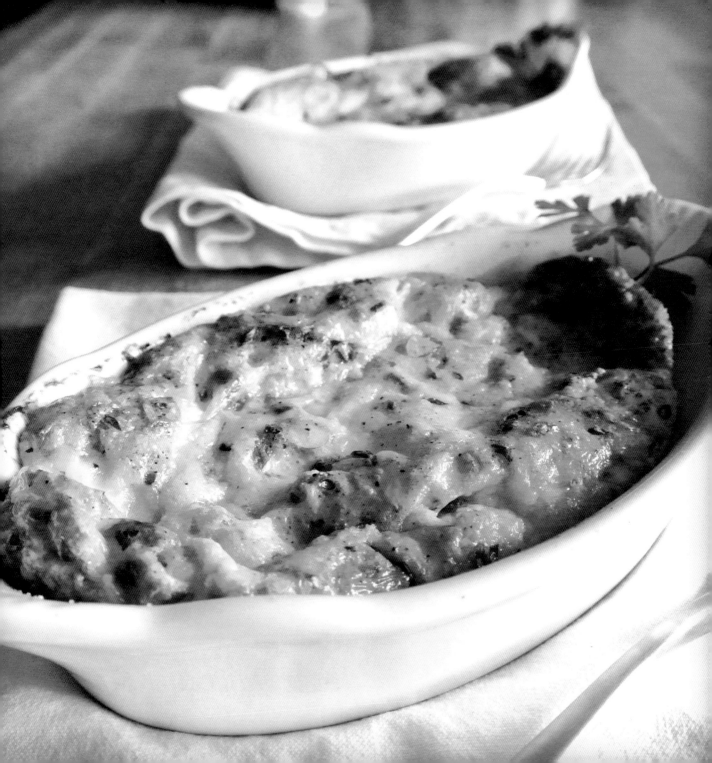

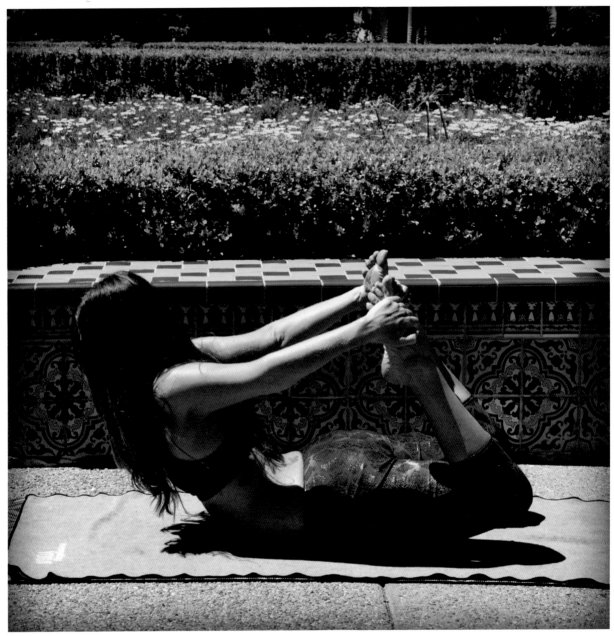

Outfit by Me and Harpua – etsy.com/shop/MeAndHarpua
Mat by Optimistic Elephant – etsy.com/shop/OptimisticElephant
Towel by Every Day Yoga – etsy.com/shop/EverydayYoga

"It is our attitude at the beginning of a difficult task which, more than anything else,
will affect its successful outcome."
– WILLIAM JAMES

BOW POSE

Begin by lying flat on your stomach with your chin on the mat and your hands resting at your sides.

On an exhalation, bend your knees. Bring your heels as close as you can to your buttocks, keeping your knees hip-distance apart.

Reach back with both hands and hold onto your outer ankles.

On an inhalation, lift your heels up toward the ceiling, drawing your thighs up and off the mat. Your head, chest, and upper torso will also lift off the mat. Draw your tailbone down firmly into the floor while you simultaneously lift your heels and thighs even higher. Lift your chest and press your shoulder blades firmly into your upper back. Draw your shoulders away from your ears and gaze forward.

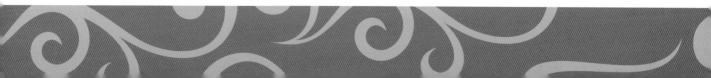

There is no excuse for skipping breakfast. It is the most important meal of the day. Make it easy with this grab-and-go healthy breakfast.

OVERNIGHT STEEL-CUT OATMEAL FOR TWO

Serves 2

2 cups boiling almond milk
½ cup steel-cut oats
⅛ teaspoon sea salt
2 tablespoons honey
½ cup applesauce
½ teaspoon cinnamon
¼ teaspoon nutmeg

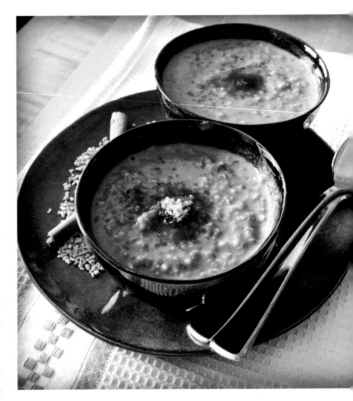

You will need 2 mason jars. Add 1 cup boiling almond milk, ¼ cup steel-cut oats, and salt to each mason jar. Cover with lids and shake. Let stand overnight. If you can, give them a shake or two when you think about it.

The next morning, shake, remove the lids, and add honey and applesauce divided between both jars. Heat in microwave for 5 minutes or reheat over the stove for 5 minutes.

Top with cinnamon and nutmeg. Add fruit or coconut sugar (like I did) if desired and serve. You can also just eat it right out of the jar if you are pressed for time.

BRIDGE POSE

Lay on your back. Bend your knees, soles of your feet parallel on the mat, as close to buttocks as possible. Inhale.

On an exhale, press your feet and arms into the mat, and then lift your hips up towards the ceiling, keeping your thighs and feet parallel.

Roll one shoulder under and then the other, bringing shoulder blades together for support. You may have to shimmy back and forth to get your shoulders all the way back.

Clasp your hands under your back and straighten your arms. Lift your hips higher. Try not to scrunch your neck as you lift your hips.

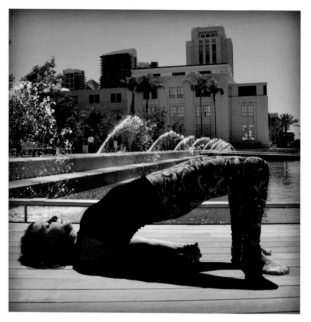

Top by Be Present – bepresent.com
Leggings by Fractal9 – etsy.com/shop/fractal9.com

"Keep away from people who try to belittle your ambitions. Small people always do that, but the really great make you feel that you, too, can become great."
– ATTRIBUTED TO MARK TWAIN

This is one of my favorite meals to throw together when I have company. It takes 20 minutes and is a healthy comfort food.

SUPER SIMPLE PAD THAI

Serves 4

14 ounces rice noodles
1 pound chicken breast, sliced thin diagonally
¾ cup Healthy Thai Peanut Sauce (page 180), divided
1 tablespoon sesame oil
5-ounce can of bamboo shoots, rinsed and drained
5-ounce can of water chestnuts, rinsed and drained
4 green onions, sliced
4 tablespoons crushed peanuts for topping

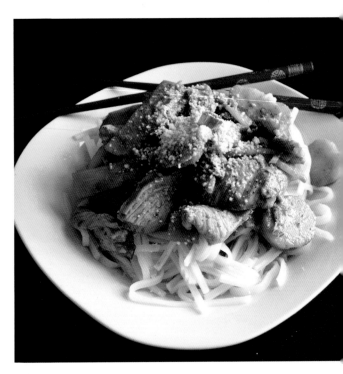

Bring 4 cups water to a boil in a large saucepan. Remove from heat. Add rice noodles; let stand for 8–10 minutes or until noodles are soft but firm. Drain and rinse under cold water. Set aside.

In a large bowl, add sliced chicken and ¼ cup of the Thai peanut sauce. Stir well to coat.

Heat a large skillet over medium-high heat. Add sesame oil and coated chicken. Cook until cooked through. Time will vary depending on how thick you cut your chicken. Mine took 5 minutes.

Top with bamboo shoots, water chestnuts, and remaining sauce. Serve over rice noodles and top with green onions and crushed peanuts.

CAMEL POSE

Begin by kneeling. Lengthen your spine and bend backwards, placing your hands on your heels.

Elongate your neck and curl your head backwards.

Slide your hands to the soles of your feet

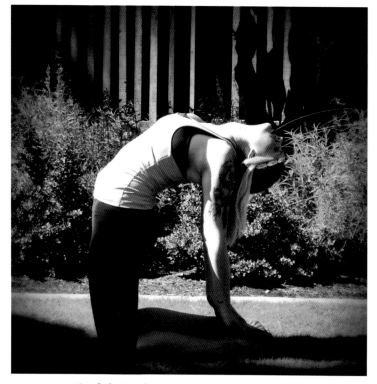

Outfit by Hotdrop Apparel – hotdropapparel.com
Headband by Pluma Crafts – etsy.com/shop/PlumaCrafts

"Life must be lived as play."
- ADAPTED FROM PLATO

CHEDDAR AND CAULIFLOWER QUICHE WITH QUINOA CRUST

Serves 6

1 cup quinoa
2 tablespoons olive oil
1 red onion, diced
1 tablespoon chopped garlic
3 cups Swiss chard or kale, roughly chopped
2 cups cauliflower florets
1 cup sharp cheddar cheese
12 eggs
2 cups milk
2 tablespoons fresh thyme leaves
½ teaspoon sea salt
black pepper to taste
¼ cup Parmesan cheese

Preheat the oven to 350 degrees F. Rinse the quinoa well and set aside to drain. Heat the oil in a pan over medium heat. Add the onion and garlic and sauté until the onion begins to brown. Add the Swiss chard and cauliflower and sauté for 1 minute, then turn off the heat and cool slightly.

Transfer the mixture to a lightly greased 9 × 13–inch baking dish and spread evenly. Top with cheddar cheese.

In a large bowl, combine the eggs, milk, thyme, salt, pepper, and rinsed quinoa and whisk until thoroughly combined. Pour immediately over the cheese-topped vegetable mixture.

Bake the casserole in the oven for 40 minutes. Remove the casserole from the oven and sprinkle the Parmesan on top. Return to oven and bake for 5 more minutes to melt the Parmesan. Let rest for 10 minutes before you serve.

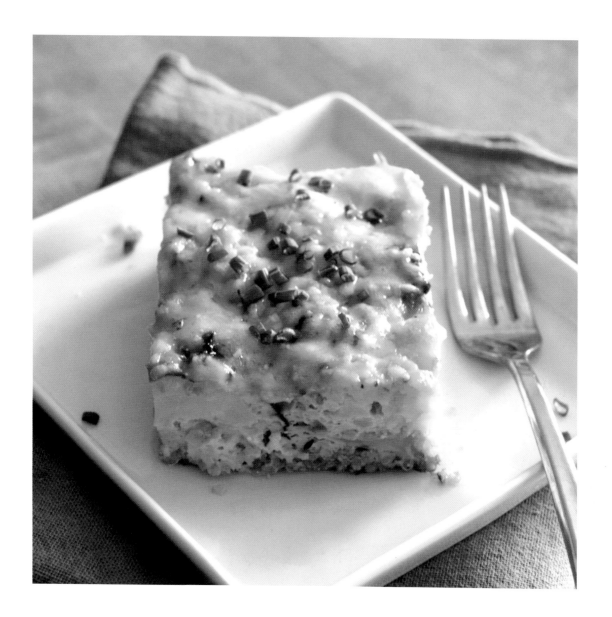

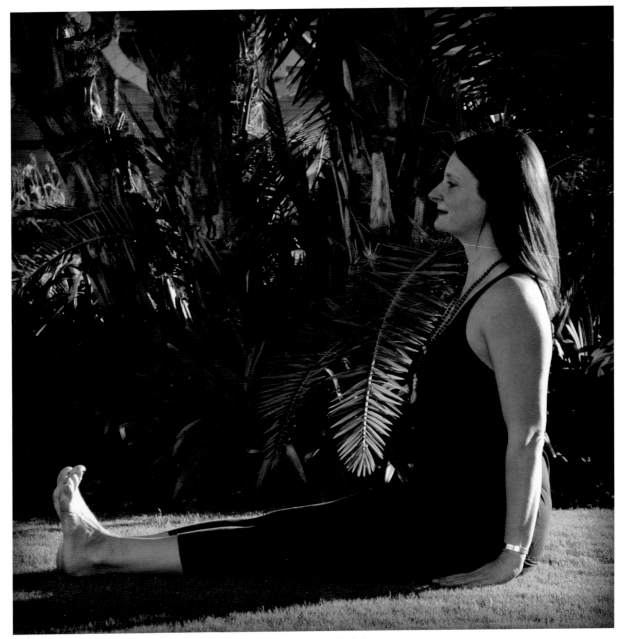

Outfit by LVR Fashion – lvrfashion.com
Necklace by True Nature Jewelry – etsy.com/shop/TrueNatureJewelry
Bracelet by Indo Love – etsy.com/shop/Indolove

STAFF POSE

Begin by sitting on the floor with your legs extended out in front of you. Sit forward on your sit bones and draw your thighs to the floor. Flex your feet and press out through your heels. Keep your big toes, inner heels, and inner knees together.

Strongly engage your thigh muscles around your thigh bones and activate the muscles surrounding your knee-caps. Press your thigh bones firmly down into the floor. Make sure your legs do not rotate outward.

Stretch your heels away from your body and tilt your pelvis slightly forward, extending the distance between your heel bones and sit bones.

Do not collapse your lower back. Work to lift your torso up from the base of your pelvis. Keep your weight evenly distributed across both sit bones.

Place your hands on the floor alongside your hips, pressing through your palms with your fingers pointing forward.

Broaden across your collarbones and lift your chest. Then, broaden across your shoulders. Draw your belly button in toward your spine. Anchor your body through your tailbone and sit tall.

"One of the things I learned the hard way was that it doesn't pay to get discouraged."
– LUCILLE BALL

This is my all-time favorite comfort food. I feel like I am indulging, but really it is good for me.

QUINOA AND BLACK BEAN ENCHILADA BAKE

Serves 4

1 tablespoon olive oil
1 small onion, diced
3 cloves garlic, minced
1 jalapeño, seeds and ribs removed, diced
juice of 1 small lime
1 teaspoon ground cumin
1 tablespoon chili powder
⅓ cup chopped cilantro
salt and pepper to taste
1 cup Perfectly Cooked Quinoa (page 60)
1 (15-ounce) can black beans, drained and rinsed
1 cup enchilada sauce
1 cup shredded Mexican cheese
optional: top with plain Greek yogurt and guacamole

Preheat the oven to 350 degrees F. Grease a medium baking dish with cooking spray and set aside.

In a large skillet, heat the tablespoon of olive oil over medium-high heat. Add the onion, garlic, and jalapeño. Sauté until softened, about 5 minutes. Add the lime juice, cumin, chili powder, and cilantro. Stir to combine. Season with salt and pepper to taste.

In a large bowl, add the cooked quinoa and black beans. Add the sautéed vegetable mixture and stir to combine. Pour in the enchilada sauce and stir. Add ½ cup shredded cheese.

Pour the black bean and quinoa mixture into the prepared baking dish. Top with remaining shredded cheese. Cover with foil, and then place in the oven. Bake for 20 minutes, then remove foil. Bake an additional 10 minutes, or until the cheese is melted and edges are bubbling. Remove from the oven and let cool for 10 minutes. Garnish with toppings, if desired. Serve warm.

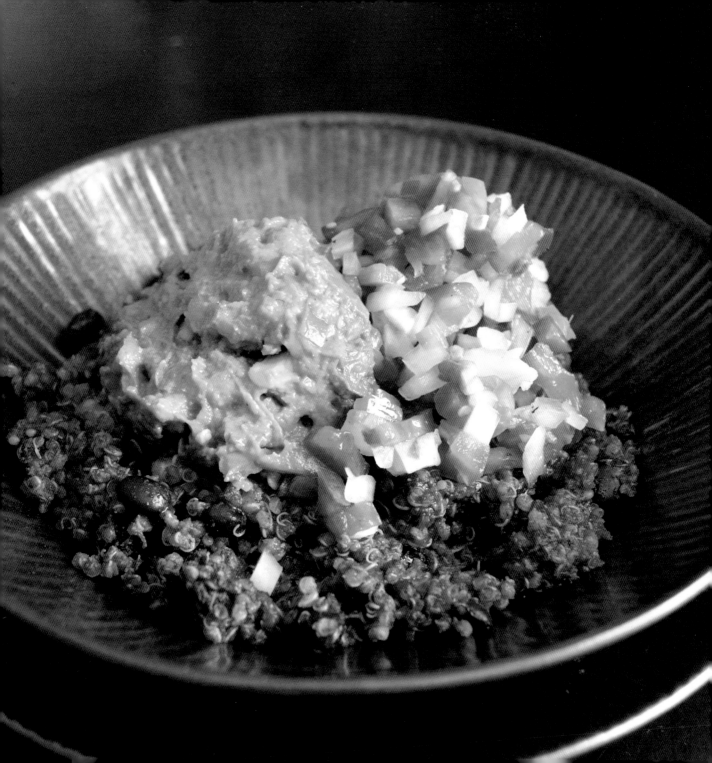

Subbing quinoa for rice kicks the nutrients up on your sushi. It tastes so good, you'll never go back to rice.

GARLIC BUTTER SHRIMP AND QUINOA SUSHI

Serves 4

FOR THE QUINOA:
2 cups cooked quinoa
⅓ cup rice vinegar
2 tablespoons agave nectar

FOR THE ROLLS:
your favorite veggies (I used 1 zucchini, 1 green pepper, 1 carrot, and chives)
4 nori sheets (dried seaweed)
4 tablespoons cream cheese or creamed Kefir cheese
soy sauce or Bragg's amino acids for dipping
pickled ginger
wasabi

SPECIAL EQUIPMENT:
bamboo sushi mat (these are pretty affordable in most kitchen stores)

Combine the cooked quinoa with the vinegar and agave. Fold gently and let it sit 5 minutes.

Cover a bamboo sushi mat with plastic wrap. Prepare the vegetables and slice into matchsticks. Place a nori sheet rough-side up on the mat. Moisten your hands and scoop ¼ of the quinoa onto the nori. Press the quinoa to spread it evenly over ¾ of the nori sheet.

Add the filling. Arrange a few pieces each of the veggies you chose in a pile in the lower third of the sheet.

It's OK if the vegetables hang over the edges of the nori. Add 1 tablespoon of the cream cheese. Roll the sushi. Roll the sushi away from you with your hands, tucking in the vegetables as you go. Press the roll into a compact rectangular log, using the mat to help you.

Slice the roll. Cut the sushi roll into 6 pieces.

Repeat with the remaining nori, quinoa, and vegetables. Serve with soy sauce, pickled ginger, and wasabi.

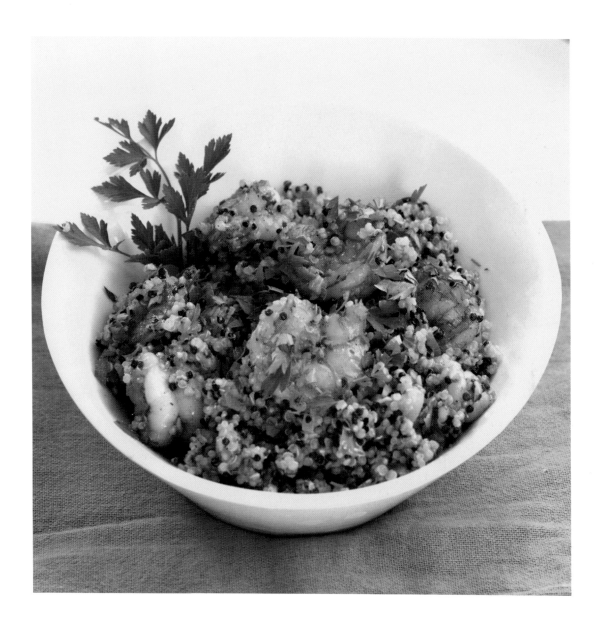

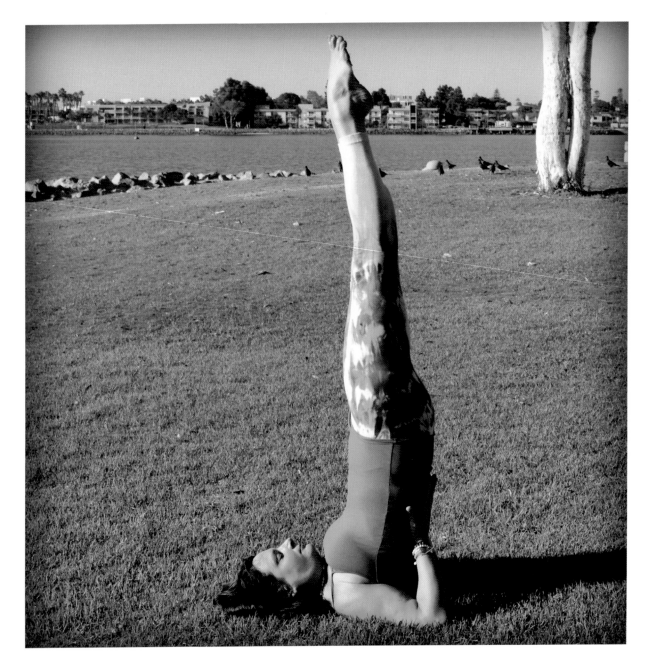

Top By Kaya Yogawear – etsy.com/shop/Kayayogawear
Leggings by Metta Body – etsy.com/shop/MettaBody

"There are two primary choices in life: to accept conditions as they exist, or accept the responsibility for changing them."
– DENIS WAITLEY

SHOULDER STAND

Begin by lying flat on your back with your legs extended and your arms at your sides, palms down. Bend your knees and place the soles of your feet flat on the floor.

On an inhalation, use your abdominal muscles to lift your legs and hips off the floor. Curl your torso and bring your knees in toward your face. Then, lift your hips and bring your torso perpendicular to the floor.

Bend your elbows and place your hands on your lower back with your fingertips pointing up toward the ceiling. Keep your elbows on the ground, shoulder-width apart. Do not let your elbows splay out to the sides.

When you are comfortable, lift your thighs so they are vertical to the floor, keeping your knees bent. Draw your tailbone toward your pubic bone. Then, straighten your legs fully and reach your feet up to the ceiling. Lift through the balls of your feet.

Try to bring your shoulders, hips, and feet into one line. Keep your head and neck in line with your spine; do not turn your head. Draw your shoulder blades firmly into your upper back. Keep a space between your chin and chest and soften your throat.

You don't need the high-calorie noodles to enjoy pad thai. Using raw ingredients typically found in pad thai, you can make a great Thai-inspired salad.

RAW PAD THAI SALAD

Serves 2

8 ounces baby spinach
1 small sweet onion
11 ounces asparagus
1 green pepper
2 green onions
½ bunch cilantro
Healthy Pad Thai Dressing (page 176)
crushed cashew nuts or peanuts for garnish

Wash and prepare all vegetables. Everything needs to be thinly sliced, grated, or cut julienne style.

Toss all ingredients to combine them.

Pour the dressing over the salad ingredients and toss well to coat the ingredients evenly. Chop the cashew nuts coarsely and either scatter the on top of the salad or offer them separately.

"There are two things a person should never be angry at—what they can help, and what they cannot."
- ATTRIBUTED TO PLATO

PLOW POSE

Begin by lying flat on your back with your legs extended and your arms at your sides, palms down. On an inhalation, use your abdominal muscles to lift your legs and hips up toward the ceiling. Bring your torso perpendicular to the floor. Straighten your legs and slowly lower your toes to the floor with your legs fully extended.

If your feet rest comfortably, extend your arms along the floor and interlace your fingers. Press your upper arms firmly into the floor, drawing down through the pinkie finger side of your hands. Align your hips over your shoulders.

Lift your tailbone higher and draw your inner groin deep into your pelvis. Keep a space between your chin and chest, and at the same time, lift your chest to open the upper back. Soften your throat.

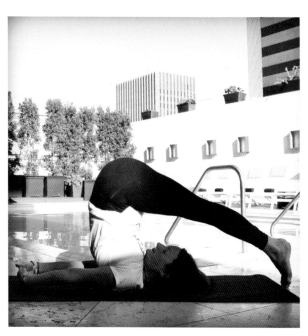

Top by My Positive Vibes – mypositivevibes.com
Leggings by DOV – dovclothing.com

This salad tastes like a yummy bowl of pasta, but is wholesome and vegan-friendly.

RAW VEGAN CAPRESE

Serves 2

3 zucchinis
2 tomatoes
1 avocado
⅛ cup balsamic vinegar
garlic salt

Peel your zucchini. You can then use a spiral cutter or a mandoline to cut the zucchini into noodles. If you do not have one, you can use a peeler and just keep peeling the zucchini long after the skin is gone. This will give it a noodle-like texture. Place zucchini noodles in a large bowl.

Dice your tomato and avocado and add them to the zucchini noodles. Add balsamic and toss to coat. Season with garlic salt to your liking. Serve cold.

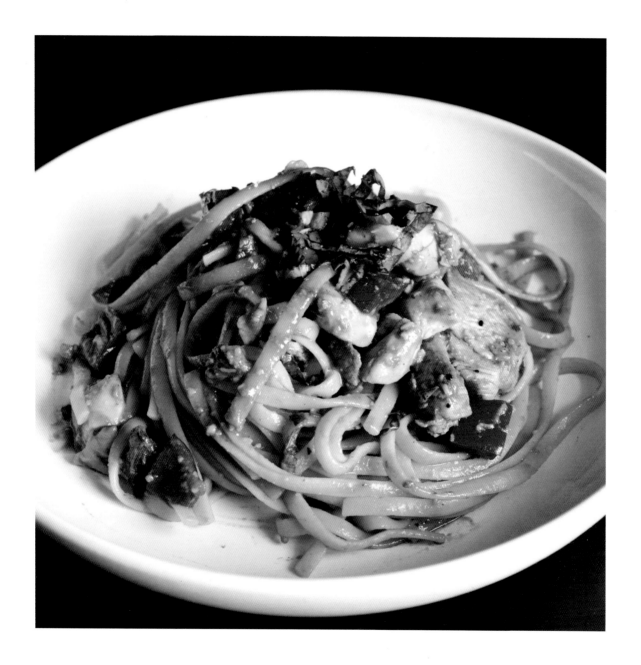

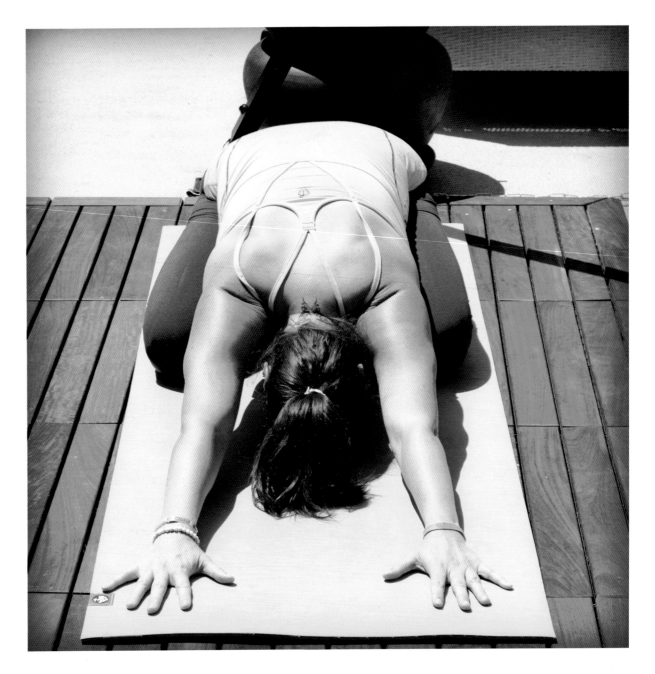

Outfit by Green Apple Active – greenappleactive.com

"The invariable mark of wisdom is to see the miraculous in the common."
– RALPH WALDO EMERSON

CHILD'S POSE

Begin on your hands and knees. Center your breath and let your thoughts begin to slow down. Turn your awareness inward.

Spread your knees wide apart while keeping your big toes touching. Rest your buttocks on your heels.

Sit up straight and lengthen your spine up through the crown of your head.

On an exhalation, bow forward, draping your torso between your thighs. Your heart and chest should rest between or on top of your thighs. Allow your forehead to come to the floor.

Keep your arms long and extended, palms facing down. Press back slightly with your hands to keep your buttocks in contact with your heels. Lengthen from your hips to your armpits, and then extend even further through your fingertips.

Let your upper back broaden. Soften and relax your lower back. Allow all tension in your shoulders, arms, and neck to drain away.

The combination of fresh herbs with high-quality full-fat spreadable Greek yogurt (Kefir) make this fish dish shine. Don't be afraid of real fat. You can use cream cheese instead, but I prefer the health benefits of Greek yogurt.

STUFFED SOLE

Serves 4

8 ounces Kefir Greek cheese cream cheese
¼ cup Parmesan cheese, plus more for dusting fish
1 tablespoon chopped dill
1 tablespoon chopped parsley
1 tablespoon chopped chives
1 tablespoon chopped oregano
1 tablespoon chopped basil
8 thinly sliced fresh wild-caught sole fillets
salt and pepper to taste

Preheat your oven to 350 degrees F. Mix your Kefir or cream cheese, Parmesan, and all the herbs and spices in a bowl.

Lay out your sole and sprinkle with salt and pepper. Spread the mixture generously on top of your fish.

Roll up your fish and place in a prepared baking dish. Sprinkle with a bit more Parmesan and salt and pepper.

Bake at 350 degrees for 35 minutes, and serve hot. I served mine over a wild rice medley with green beans on the side. It was lovely.

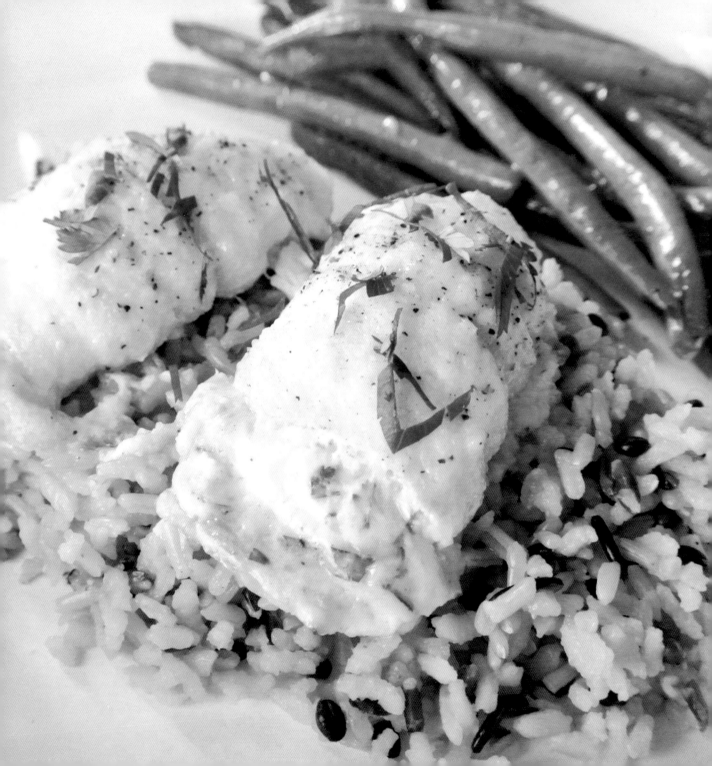

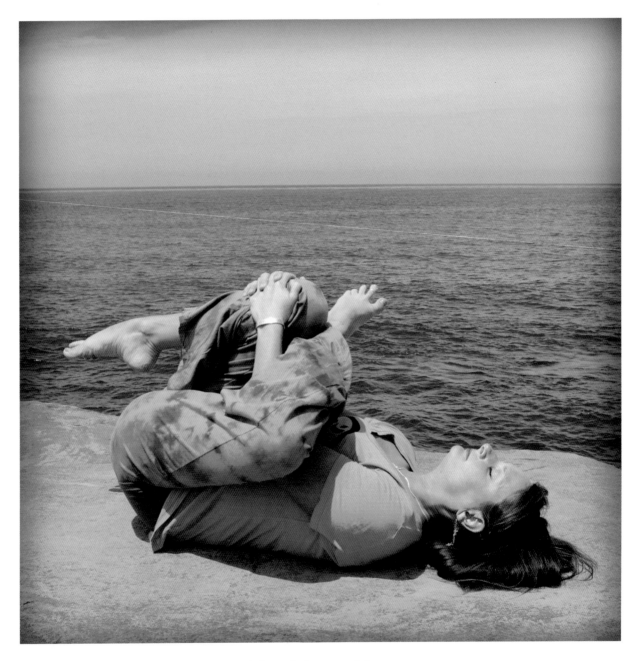

Outfit by Soul Flower – soul-flower.com
Bracelet by Indo Love – etsy.com/shop/IndoLove

> "There are only two ways to live your life. One is as though nothing is a miracle. The other is as though everything is a miracle."
> **– ALBERT EINSTEIN**

EYE OF THE NEEDLE POSE

Lie on your back, knees bent, soles of your feet on the floor. Breathe deeply and let the body relax into the mat. Cross left ankle over right knee.

Bring both hands to the right shin, lifting your right foot off the floor and threading your left hand through your legs. Using your hands, draw your right thigh toward chest. Open your left hip. If this "reach through the hole around the knee" is not possible, clasp hands together around top of right knee. Try not to lift head and shoulders off of the mat.

Press your right knee away from your body gently while drawing left knee to chest. Hold pose for 6–24 breaths, release hands, and bring soles of your feet to the mat. Repeat on the other side.

This salad is full of nutrients that you may not think to put together, but once you combine these flavors your taste buds will be very happy!

THAI CHICKEN SALAD

Serves 4

FOR THE SALAD:
3 cups coleslaw mix
1 mango, peeled and chopped
1 cucumber, cubed
1 cup bok choy, chopped
4 cups cooked chicken breasts, shredded or cut in small pieces

FOR THE DRESSING:
juice from 2 limes
2 tablespoons olive oil
2 tablespoons Bragg's amino acids or soy sauce
2 tablespoons agave nectar
2 tablespoons peanut butter or almond butter
1 teaspoon fish sauce
a pinch of red pepper flakes

Add all salad ingredients to a large bowl and toss.

In a smaller bowl, mix all dressing ingredients together. Pour over salad and toss well. Serve!

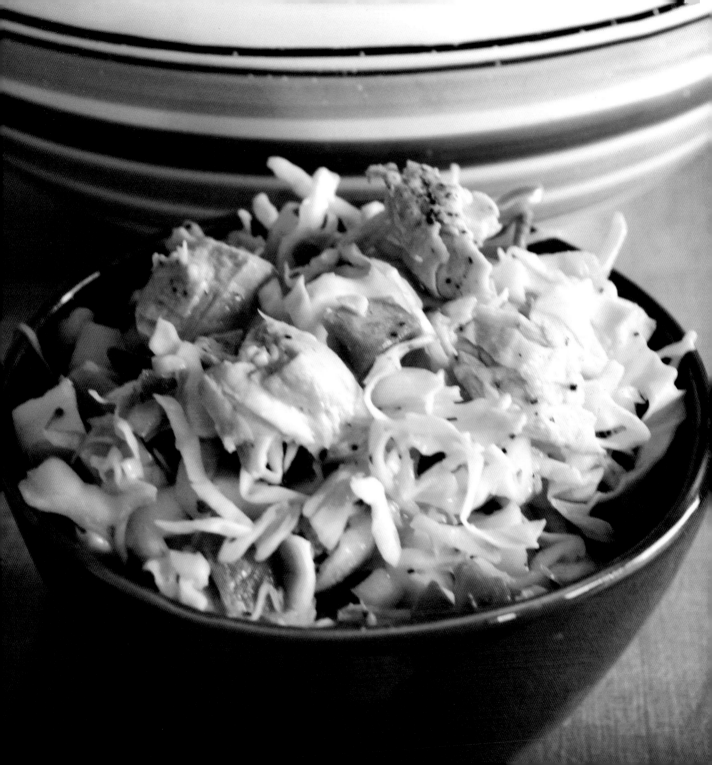

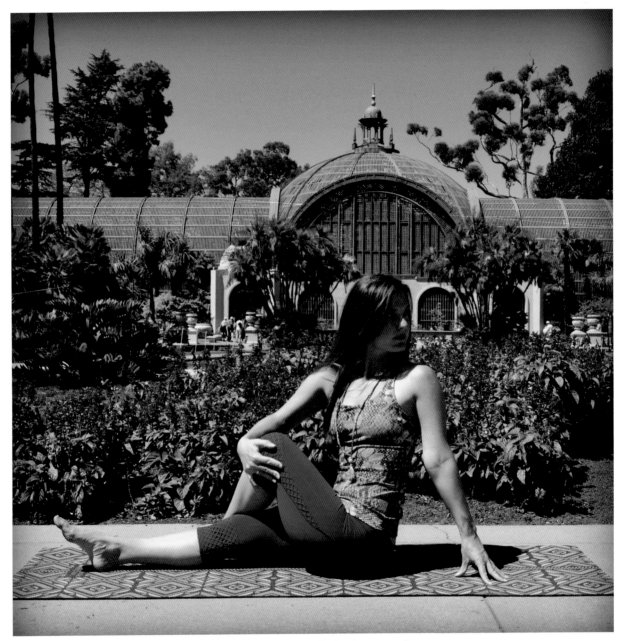

Outfit by Hotdrop Apparel – hotdropapparel.com
Necklace by True Nature Jewelry – etsy.com/shop/TrueNatureJewelry
Mat by Optimistic Elephant – etsy.com/shop/OptimisticElephant

> "We don't see things as they are; we see them as we are."
> **- ANONYMOUS**

HALF LORD OF THE FISHES POSE

Sit down on mat; stretch right leg out in front as pelvis is pressed firmly on the mat. Cross left leg over your right leg, left foot resting flat on mat next to right knee.

Bend right leg, bringing right heel next to left hip. Pull left knee towards your chest with your right hand.

Exhale. Twist your trunk towards the back with head facing backward, and place your left hand on the mat next to your left hip.

There is no way that anyone can walk away from eating a bowl of this chili and still feel like they need meat. You are left full and satisfied. You can spice it up or spice it down by managing the amount of peppers you put in.

VEGETARIAN/VEGAN CHILI

Serves 4

½ large sweet onion, chopped
2 cloves garlic, minced
4 jalapeño peppers, seeded and minced
1 small bell pepper, finely chopped
1 celery stick, chopped
1 teaspoon oregano
1 tablespoon ground cumin
3 tablespoons chili powder
1 teaspoon cayenne pepper
1 teaspoon salt
½ teaspoon black pepper
2 cans kidney beans, with liquid
2 cans black beans, with liquid
1 (15-ounce) can tomato sauce
1 (29-ounce) can puréed tomatoes

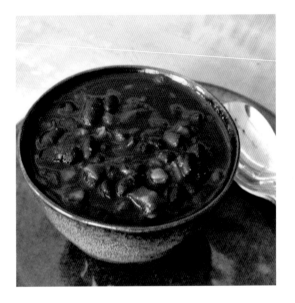

In a large stock pot, add in the onion, garlic, jalapeños, bell pepper, and celery and mix this together.

Add the rest of the ingredients and bring it to a boil. Once it boils, reduce the heat and let it simmer for 1 hour.

EAR PRESSURE POSE

From Shoulder Stand (page 143), slowly bend your knees down towards your forehead.

Separate your knees and lower them down toward the ground. Squeeze your ears gently with the insides of your knees and release your hands to the ground, palms facing down.

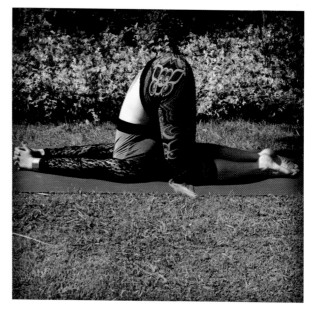

Outfit by ProperFit – etsy.com/shop/ProperFit
Cuff by Indo Love – etsy.com/shop/IndoLove
Mat by Manduka – manduka.com

"You alone are the judge of your worth and your goal is to discover infinite worth in yourself, no matter what anyone else thinks."
– DEEPAK CHOPRA

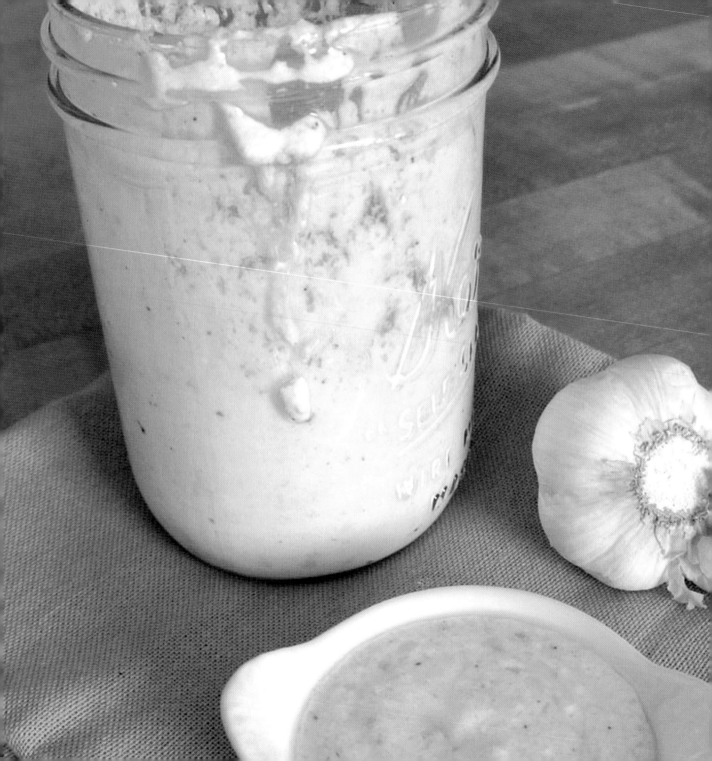

SECRET SAUCES

I keep a bunch of sauces and dressings on hand for extra flavor and added nutrients. They are the extra kick a lot of my recipes use. I am now revealing them to you so you can enjoy eating healthy while feeling like you are indulging.

This caramel sauce is a healthier way for you to enjoy a treat. Adding it in moderation will help your sweet tooth while giving you some healthy nutrients.

CARAMEL SAUCE

Makes 1 cup

1 can full-fat coconut milk
¼ cup maple syrup
¼ cup honey
pinch of salt
1 tablespoon coconut oil
2 teaspoons vanilla extract

In a large saucepan with a thick bottom, combine coconut milk, maple syrup, honey, and salt.

Bring to boil over medium-high heat. Lower the heat to medium-low and let reduce for about 50 minutes, stirring every now and then. Add coconut oil and cook for 5 minutes until it reaches a deep caramel color.

Don't rush it. The process could be faster or slower, depending on how hot your burner is. Stir every so often towards the end to keep the bottom from burning too much. Remove from the heat, transfer to a bowl, and let cool for about 5 minutes, then stir until smooth and glossy. Store in an airtight container in the fridge until you are ready to use. It keeps for 2 weeks.

> "You can tell more about a person by what he says about others than you can by what others say about him."
> **– ATTRIBUTED TO LEO AIKMAN**

PIGEON POSE

Start on hands and knees in a Tabletop Pose (see page 111).

Slide right knee up between hands so outer right leg is resting on the mat. Make sure left hip is always pointing down toward the mat. If hip begins to raise up or if knee feels stressed, draw your right foot back in toward your body. If hips are more open, inch right foot away. People who are very flexible should try to get the shin parallel to the top of the mat, but this takes years to accomplish.

Center yourself so your weight is even. Slide back knee away until right buttock reaches the floor or as low as possible. Remember to breathe. The longer you stay in this pose, the more you allow your hips to settle in and open up. Remember to always repeat on the other side.

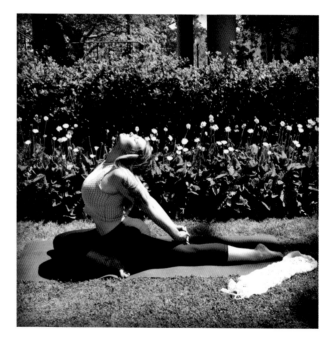

Outfit by ProperFit – etsy.com/shop/ProperFit
Crocheted mat bag by Buy Karen – etsy.com/shop/buykaren

Say goodbye to refined sugar! This all-natural sweetener goes perfect in almost every recipe. Add it to oat-meal, smoothies, yogurt, baking . . . the list goes on. Your body will love you and your taste buds will thank you. Did I mention it was easy to make and stores well? Win-win!

DATE PASTE

Makes 1 cup

1 package pitted Medjool dates (about 6 ounces, 170 grams, or 30 dates)
½ cup almond milk
1 teaspoon vanilla extract

Put all ingredients in a food processor or blender and purée until smooth. You may need to stop halfway through and scrape the sides down, then proceed with blending until smooth.

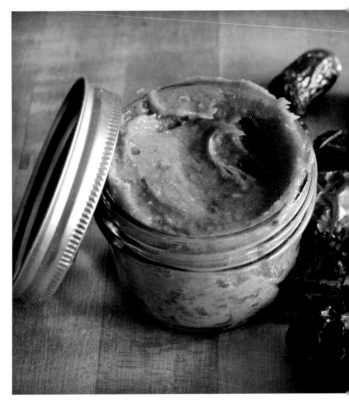

SHOELACE POSE

Kneel on all fours, then place one knee behind the other and sit back between the heels. Try to keep one knee stacked on the other as best you can.

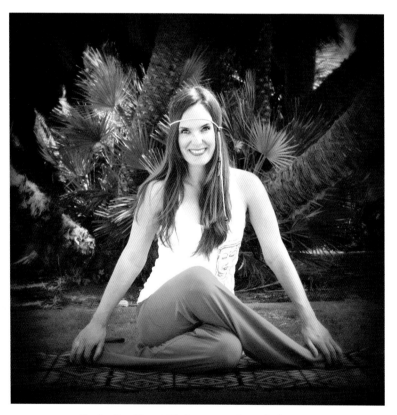

Top by Om Shanti Clothing – omshanticlothing.com
Pants by Hyde Organic – yogahyde.com
Headband by Pluma Crafts – etsy.com/shop/PlumaCrafts

So many people get it twisted by ordering a salad and then topping it with high-calorie, mayonnaise-filled dressing. Using Greek yogurt truly makes your salad dressing healthy.

GARLIC PARMESAN SALAD DRESSING

Makes 1 cup

3 cloves fresh garlic
4 tablespoons white vinegar
2 tablespoons grated Parmesan cheese
½ teaspoon sea salt
¼ teaspoon fresh, coarsely ground black pepper
5 tablespoons extra-virgin olive oil
½ cup Greek yogurt

Squeeze the garlic through a garlic press and into a small bowl. Measure and add in the vinegar, cheese, salt, and pepper.

Drizzle in a steady stream of olive oil while whisking. Next, add in the Greek yogurt and stir to combine. Check for seasoning before pouring the salad dressing into an airtight container and refrigerating for a few hours.

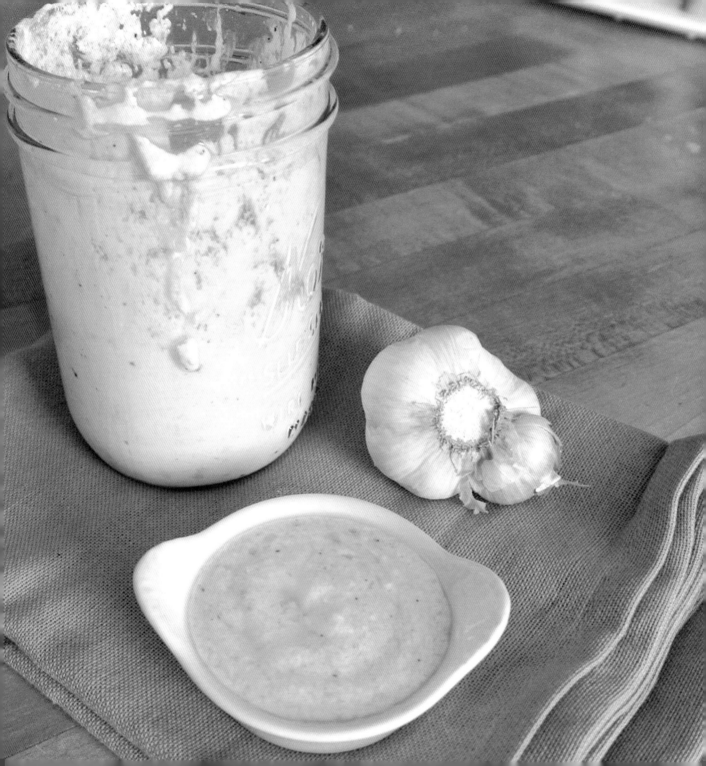

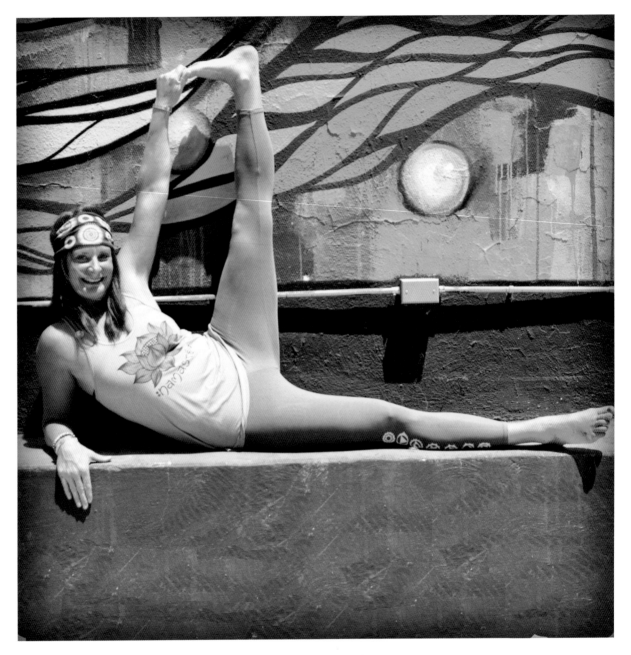

Outfit by Soul Flower – soul-flower.com

> "Your altitude, not your aptitude, will determine your altitude."
> **– ZIG ZIGLAR**

SIDE-RECLINING LEG LIFT

Lay on the floor or mat on your right side. Press actively through your right heel, flex the ankle, and use the outside of the foot to stabilize the position.

Stretch your right arm straight out along the floor, parallel to your torso, so that you create one long line from the heels to your fingertips. Bend your right elbow and support your upper body.

Externally rotate your left leg so the toes point toward the ceiling, then bend and draw the knee toward your torso. Reach across the inside of the leg and take hold of the left big toe with your index and middle fingers. Secure the grip by wrapping the thumb around the two fingers. On an inhale, extend the leg up toward the ceiling. The raised leg will likely angle slightly forward, while the top buttock will drop back. Firm the sacrum against the pelvis; this creates a kind of fulcrum that will help you move the leg slightly back into a perpendicular position.

Use on salads and sandwiches and as a dip.

GREEK DRIZZLE SAUCE

Makes 1 cup

1 cup plain Greek yogurt
½ tablespoon lemon zest
1 tablespoon freshly squeezed lemon juice
1 tablespoon salt
1 tablespoon freshly chopped cilantro leaves
2 teaspoons freshly chopped parsley leaves
½ teaspoon ground cumin

Mix ingredients together in a small bowl and chill until ready to use.

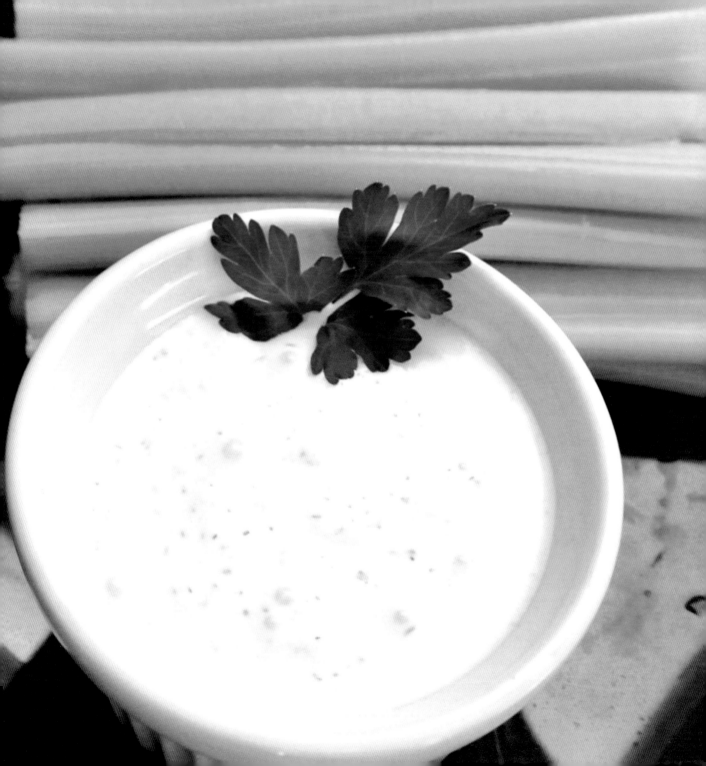

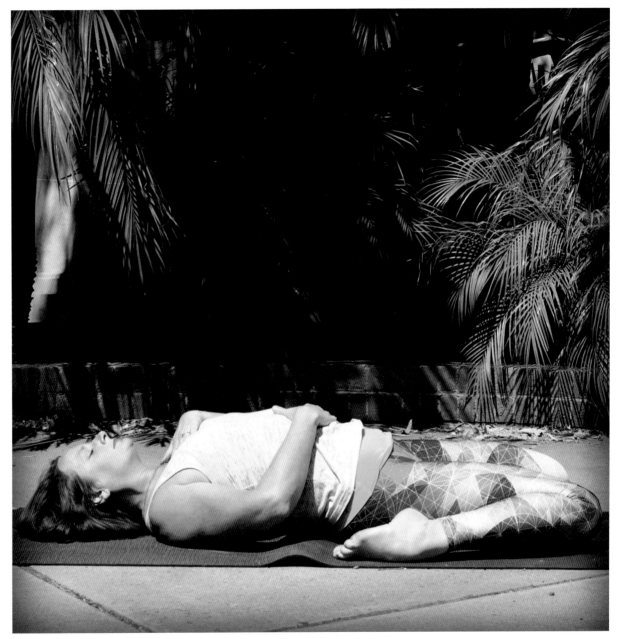

Top by Think Positive Apparel – thinkpositiveapparel.com
Leggings By Inner Fire Apparel – myinnerfire.com
Hip Wallet by Hips Sister – hipssister.com

RECLINED HERO POSE

Begin kneeling on the floor with your inner knees together and your thighs perpendicular to the floor. Open your feet slightly wider than your hips. Keep the tops of your feet flat on the floor and your big toes angled in toward each other. Press down evenly across the tops of both feet.

Exhaling, sit down between your feet. Rest your weight equally across both sit bones. Keep your feet directly in line with your shins. Do not let your feet splay wide open or turn inward.

Place your hands on the floor behind you. Lean your weight into your hands, then lower your elbows and forearms to the floor; continue to lower yourself all the way to the floor. Allow your thigh bones to release deep into your hip sockets. Beginners may have the knees slightly apart (an inch or two); those with more flexibility should keep the thighs pressing together. Do not let your knees splay wider than your hips.

You can rest your arms at your sides, or bring one hand to your heart and the other to your tummy.

HEALTHY HOISIN SAUCE

Makes ½ cup

4 tablespoons gluten-free soy sauce or Bragg's amino acids
1 tablespoon peanut butter
1 tablespoon honey
3 teaspoons white vinegar
¼ teaspoon garlic powder
2 teaspoons sesame oil
2 teaspoons sriracha chili sauce
⅛ teaspoon black pepper

Add all ingredients in a large bowl and whisk for a minute or two until well blended.

Store in an airtight container in the fridge.

"A lot of people seeking new beginnings have never finished with the past."
– BYRON PULSIFER

HERO POSE

Begin kneeling on the floor with your inner knees together and your thighs perpendicular to the floor. Open your feet slightly wider than your hips. Keep the tops of your feet flat on the floor and your big toes angled in toward each other. Press down evenly across the tops of both feet.

Exhaling, sit down between your feet. Rest your weight equally across both sit bones. Keep your feet directly in line with your shins. Do not let your feet splay wide open or turn inward.

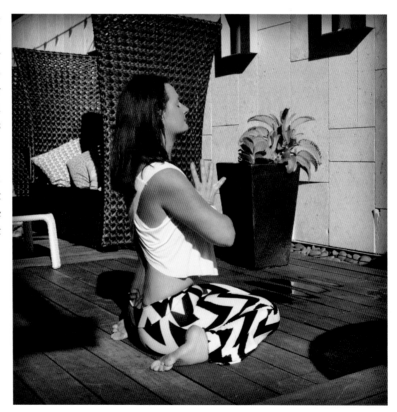

Top by Onzie – onzie.com
Pants by Liza Jane Apparel – etsy.com/shop/lizajanehandmade

HEALTHY PAD THAI DRESSING

Makes 1/2 cup

2 tablespoons olive oil
2 tablespoons apple cider vinegar
2 garlic cloves
juice and zest of 1 lime
1 teaspoon gluten-free soy sauce or Bragg's amino acids
2 pinches chili pepper
sea salt and fresh ground pepper to taste
¼ cup crushed peanuts or cashews

Mix together in a small bowl the olive oil and the vinegar. Add the garlic, stirring to blend smoothly. Stir in the lime juice, zest, soy sauce, and chili pepper. Add a little salt and pepper to taste. Stir in the crushed nuts very last.

Store in an airtight container in the fridge for up to 2 weeks.

BOAT POSE

Sit on the floor with knees bent, feet flat on the floor, and your hands on your sides. With your back straight and your head in line with your body, lift up through the chest and lean back to about a 45-degree angle.

Try to straighten the legs and keep them together, raising them as high as is comfortable. Keep neck and shoulders relaxed. Once you feel balanced, you may choose to reach the arms forward or up with palms facing each other.

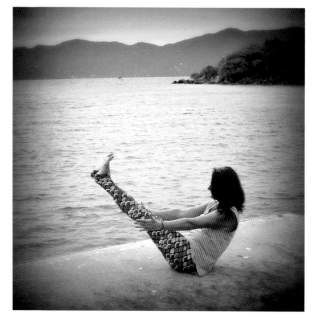

Leggings by Fractal9 – etsy.com/shop/Fractal9
Top by Green Apple Activewear – greenappleactive.com

"Beginnings are only difficult without any action."
– BYRON PULSIFER

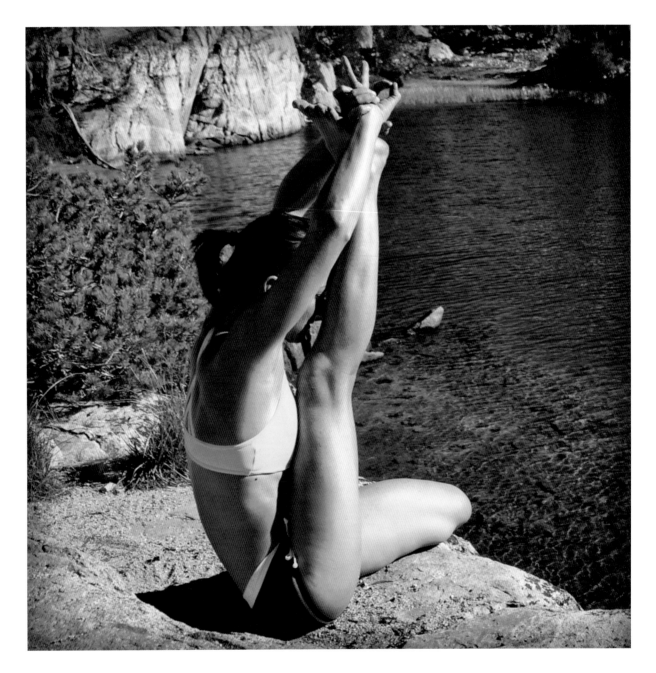

Outfit by Dragonfly – dragonfly-yogawear.com

HERON POSE

Sit in Staff Pose (page 137) with your legs outstretched in front of you. Bend your right knee and fold the right foot next to the right hip. Keep the top of the foot on the floor and the toes pointing back into Reclined Pose (page 173).

You need to be able to sit evenly on both sit bones; if not, sit on blocks or place a folded blanket under the sit bone of the straight leg. Keep the knees together.

Bend your left leg, placing the foot on the floor in front of the hip. Hold the left foot with both hands, or if impossible to straighten the left leg, hold a strap around the left foot or even the left lower leg.

On an inhalation, begin to straighten your left leg, keeping the spine long, the chest open, and the sternum lifted. Once the leg is straight, bring the leg in close to the chest and the head to the shin bone, with all the previous actions still in place.

The final (and advanced) hand position is to hold the left wrist with the right hand, around the left foot.

This sauce is a great as a dip, in pad thai, or on a salad.

HEALTHY THAI PEANUT SAUCE

Makes approximately ¾ cup

1 tablespoon sesame oil
3 cloves garlic, minced
1 tablespoon peanut butter
½ cup rice vinegar
4 tablespoons fish sauce
4 tablespoons Sucanat or coconut sugar
1 teaspoon crushed red pepper

In a small saucepan, heat sesame oil and garlic over medium heat, until fragrant (not brown).

Add remaining ingredients while stirring frequently until it reaches a boil. Remove from heat. Store in an airtight container in the fridge until use.

REVOLVED HEAD-TO-KNEE POSE

Start from a seated Staff Pose (page 137) and open your legs out as wide as is comfortable in a wide-legged straddle. Bend your right knee and bring your right sole to the inner left thigh/groin. Keep your left foot flexed.

Sit tall and elongate your spine. Lean your torso to the left, reaching with your left hand for your big toe.

Gently twist your torso away from the left leg, opening your chest to the right. Gaze upwards but do not over-rotate your neck. Raise your right arm overhead with your right biceps over your right ear. Always remember to repeat on your opposite side.

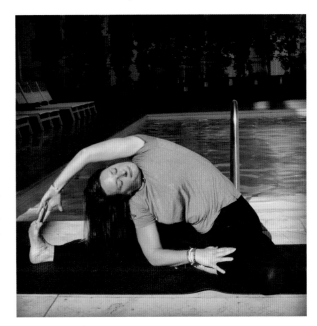

Top by Pieces to Peaces – piecestopeaces.com
Leggings by Dov Clothing – dovclothing.com
Bracelets by IndoLove – etsy.com/shop/indolove

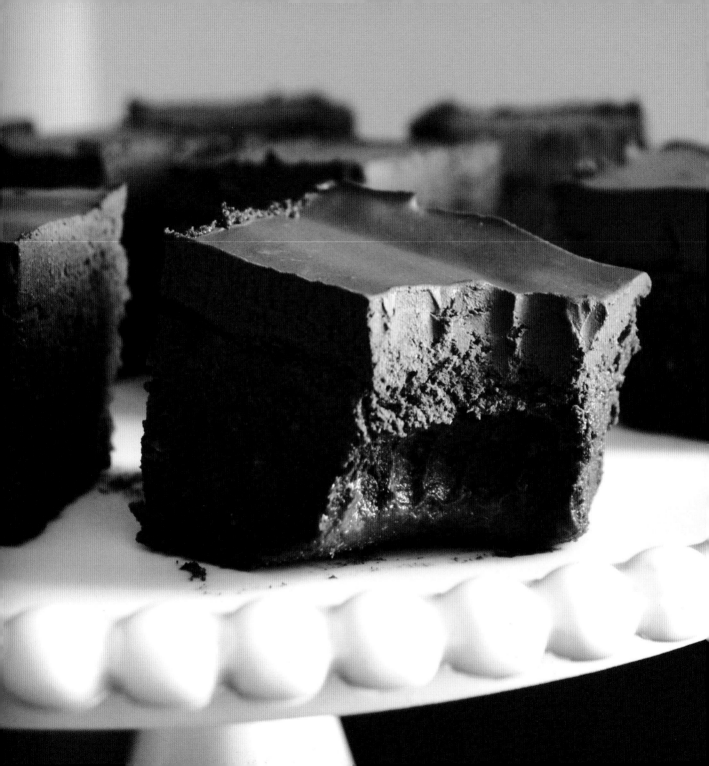

HEALTHY SWEET TREATS

Everyone needs a treat. With these wholesome recipes, you can eat treats for breakfast. They taste even better than the sugar-filled treats you are used to. Don't believe me? Give these recipes a try!

These protein cookies are raw, vegan, gluten-free, and dairy-free. Yet they taste like you are eating a sinful dessert. The cookies are a delicious blend of unsweetened fruits, nuts, and spices

APPLE PIE COOKIES

Makes 12 cookies

¾ cup dried organic apple slices
¼ cup organic Medjool dates, pitted
½ cup almonds
½ cup walnuts
½ teaspoon cinnamon

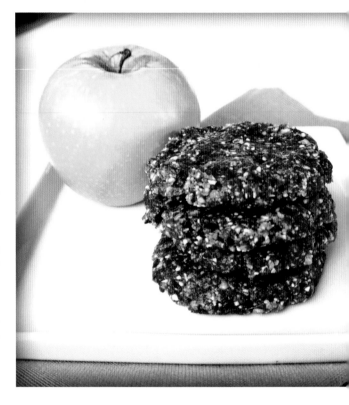

Soak the dried apples in warm water for 5–10 minutes. Meanwhile, gather remaining ingredients and pour into a food processor.

Drain the fruit and add to the food processor. Process for 30–60 seconds or until the mixture sticks together when pinched with your fingers.

Roll into balls and then flatten on parchment paper. Store in the fridge for up to 2 weeks in an airtight container. Store in the freezer for up to 3 months.

LOTUS POSE

Begin in a seated Staff Pose (page 137). Lift your right knee and hug it to your chest. Then, bring your right ankle to the crease of your left hip so the sole of your right foot faces the sky. The top of your foot should rest on your hip crease.

Next, bend your left knee. Cross your left ankle over the top of your right shin. The sole of your left foot should also face upwards, and the top of your foot and ankle should rest on your hip crease.

Draw your knees as close together as possible. Press your groin toward the floor, sit up straight, and bring your hands to prayer position.

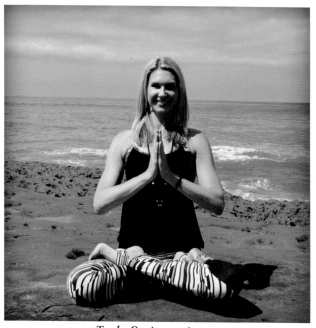

Top by Onzie – onzie.com
Pants by Proper Fit – etsy.com/shop/properfit
Necklace by True Nature Jewelry – etsy.com/shop/TrueNatureJewelry

Who doesn't love a good banana bread? It is so tempting, but so full of calories and processed sugar and flour. These cookies are suitable for breakfast, consisting of fruit and nuts. They make a great on-the-go snack. I make up a batch and grab one on the way out the door. 140 wholesome calories in each cookie. (One piece of toast has 120 calories).

HEALTHY BANANA BREAD COOKIES

Makes 12 cookies

1 cup pitted Medjool dates
½ cup dried banana
1 cup raw almonds
½ teaspoon pure vanilla extract
1 teaspoon cinnamon

Add all ingredients to your food processor and process until a dough forms.

Roll 2 tablespoons of dough into a ball and press it flat into a cookie on parchment.

Store in an airtight container in the freezer; they stay fresh for months.

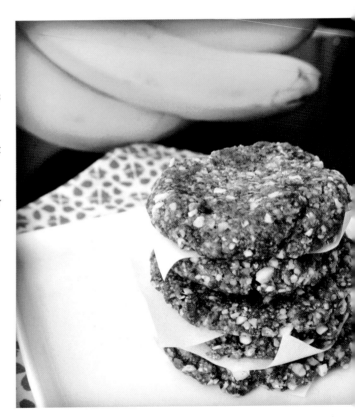

LIFTED LOTUS

Sit on the ground with your head and spine erect. Extend your legs forward such that your knees and heels are placed together. With the help of your hands, place your right foot on the left thigh and then your left foot on the right thigh. This is the Lotus Pose (page 185).

Place your palms on the ground next to your hips. Gradually and smoothly raise your body above ground level so that your entire body weight rests on the palms of your hands.

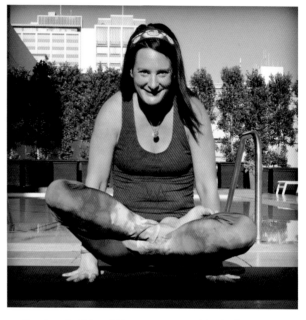

Leggings by Schatzi Brown – etsy.com/shop/SchatziBrown
Necklace by The Run Home – etsy.com/shop/TheRunHome
Headband by Soul Flower – soul-flower.com

"Finish each day and be done with it. You have done what you could. Some blunders and absurdities no doubt crept in; forget them as soon as you can. Tomorrow is a new day. You shall begin it serenely and with too high a spirit to be encumbered with your old nonsense."
– RALPH WALDO EMERSON

I love to have these in the morning for an extra boost of protein and coffee.

RAW, VEGAN, GLUTEN-FREE CAFFÉ MOCHA COOKIES

Makes 12 cookies

1 cup almonds
¼ cup walnuts
¼ cup cashews
2 tablespoons cocoa powder
1 tablespoons ground coffee beans
1½ cup Medjool dates, pitted

Start out by adding nuts to your food processor. Pulse until the nuts resemble bread crumbs.

Add cocoa powder and ground coffee beans and process until well blended. Add your dates and process until the dates have puréed and fully blended with the nuts. The dough should look like thick batter.

Roll the dough into 2-tablespoon rolls and then squish flat to make a cookie. I do this on parchment paper. Place the flattened cookies in the freezer for 10 minutes to set. Then serve. I store mine in an airtight container in the freezer until I serve them. They last for months in the freezer.

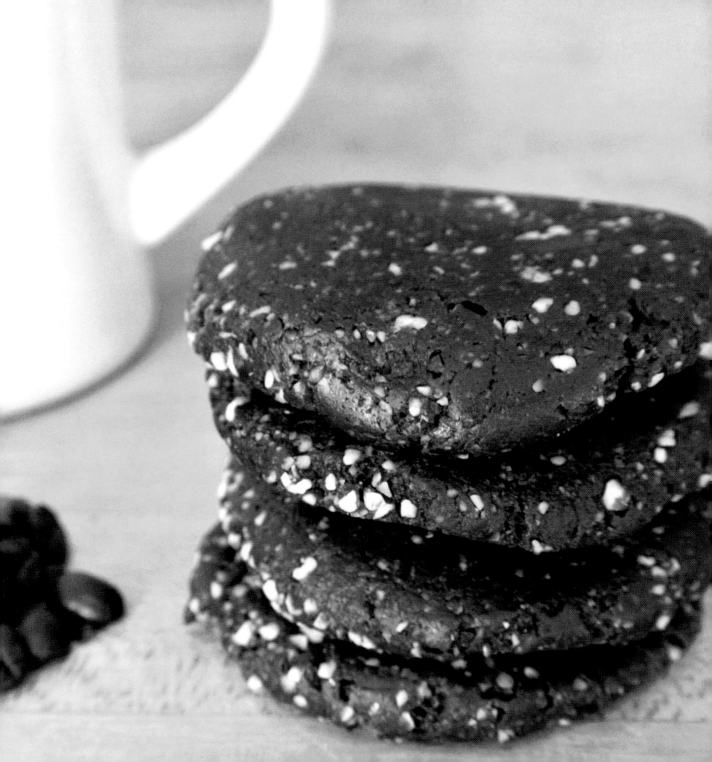

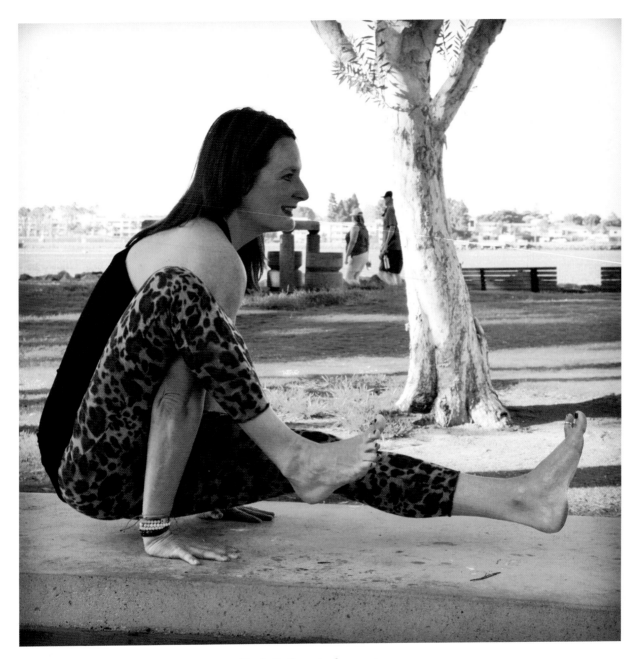

Top by Be Present – bepresent.com
Pants by Liza Jane Apparel – etsy.com/shop/lizajanehandmade

ELEPHANT'S TRUNK POSE

Begin in Staff Pose (page 137). Lift your right shin off the floor with your hands. Cradle the lower leg in your arms, keeping the shin roughly parallel with the floor. Place your right knee in the crook of your right elbow and your right foot in the crook of your left elbow. Make sure to flex the right foot and try to keep sitting up straight and tall. Avoid rounding the spine forward or leaning too far backward.

Rock the cradled right leg gently back and forth in the hip socket to loosen up your hip.

Release the right arm from the right knee. Thread the right arm under the right knee, placing the right hand on the ground just outside the right buttock. Keep the right arm bent at the elbow and the back of your right knee resting on your upper arm.

You can use your left hand on the right foot to work the right calf as close as possible to the right shoulder. The back of your right thigh will be on the back of your right upper arm. The higher up you can get the calf on your arm, the smoother the rest of the pose will be.

Straighten and extend the left leg on the floor in front of you. Release the left arm and place your left hand on the floor outside the left thigh. Your two hands should be parallel.

Press into both palms and lift your buttocks and left leg off the floor. As you get stronger, eventually you will be able to lift up on your fingers.

I make up a big batch of these ahead of time and keep them in the freezer for quick grab-and-go snacks. They go great with your morning coffee or tea and provide enough energy to keep you going until lunch.

HEALTHY CHOCOLATE BROWNIE COOKIES

Makes 12 cookies

¼ cup walnuts
½ cup whole almonds
¼ cup unsweetened cocoa powder
1¾ cups Medjool dates, pitted

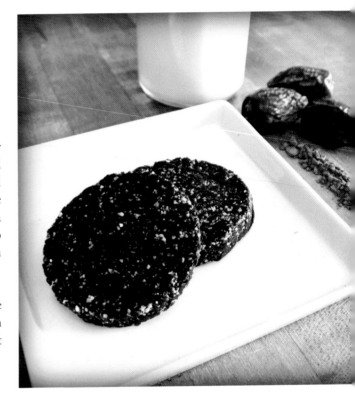

Put your walnuts and almonds in a food processor and pulse until the nuts resemble bread crumbs. Add your cocoa powder and pulse a few times until well blended. Next, add your pitted dates. Process until the dates have been broken down and you are left with a gooey batter. Roll into a ball and press your batter into a cookie. Place them on parchment paper and put in the fridge for 20 minutes to set.

Store in an airtight container or freezer bag in the freezer or fridge. I keep mine in the freezer and then pack them in my husband's lunch, and they are soft and gooey again for him by lunchtime.

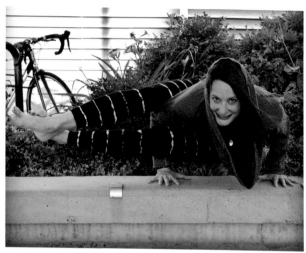

Outfit by LVR Fashion – lvrfashion.com
Necklace by The Run Home – therunhome.com

"Whatever you do, or dream you can, begin it. Boldness has genius
and power and magic in it."
– ATTRIBUTED TO JOHANN WOLFGANG VON GOETHE

8-ANGLE POSE

Sit and hug your right knee in toward your chest with your arms. If there's room, press the bottom of your right foot into your left elbow, wrap your right arm around your right knee and shin, and join your hands to cradle the leg. Lengthen your torso and sit up tall. Relax your shoulders downward. Sway your leg from side to side to open your hips.

Once your hips feel open, hook your right hand under your right calf and bring your right leg and the underside of your knee to rest on top of your right shoulder.

Cross your left ankle over your right. Put your right shoulder underneath your right knee. With both of your hands on the ground shoulder-distance apart, start to bend your elbows as you squeeze your legs together on your right upper arm.

Reach your chest forward as your weight transfers into your hands, pressing deep into your fingertips. Remember to repeat on the other side!

I used to crave soft serve all the time until I came up with this solution. It curbs my sweet tooth and rich creamy cravings in one dip.

CHOCOLATE GREEK YOGURT DIP

Serves 1

½ cup plain Greek yogurt
3 tablespoons cocoa powder
1 teaspoon stevia
½ teaspoon vanilla
fresh fruit (for dipping)

Combine all ingredients in a medium-sized bowl. Stir until it is an even dark color and all of the stevia has dissolved, about 3 minutes. Serve with fresh fruit for dipping.

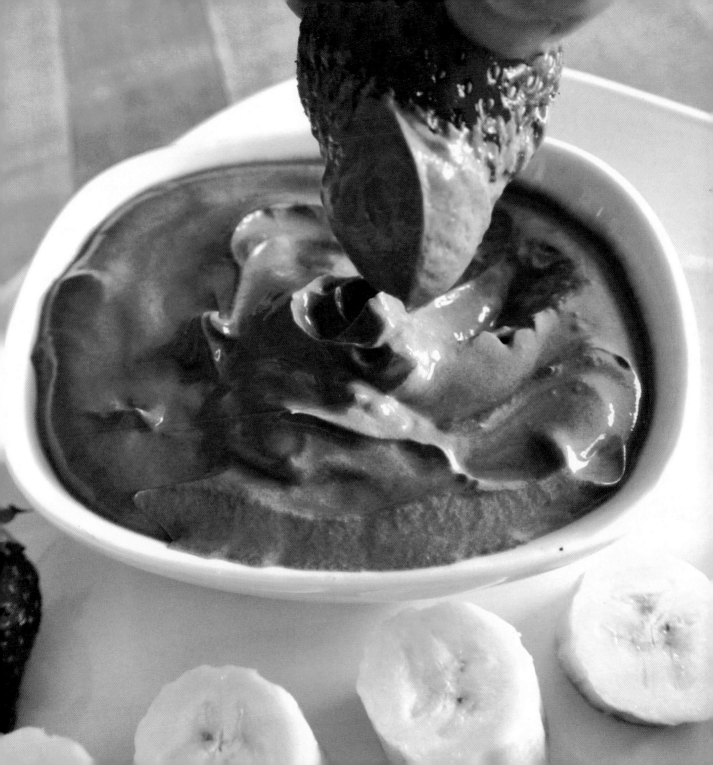

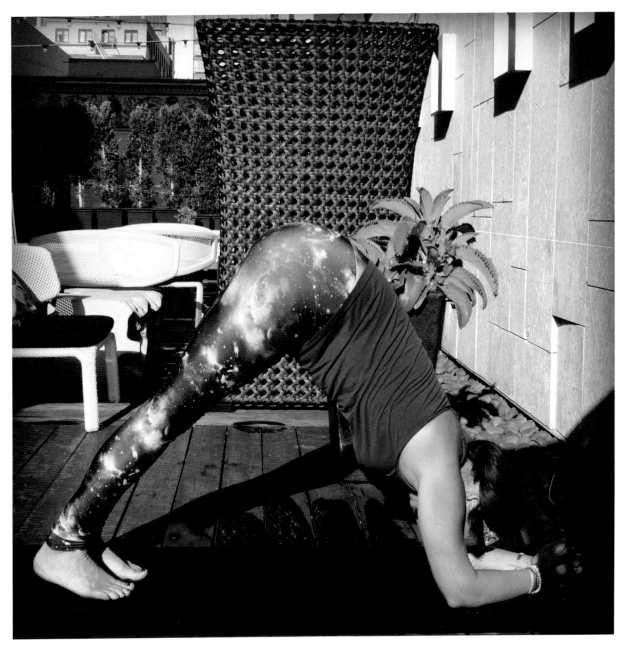

Top by Be Present – bepresent.com
Leggings by Fractal9 – etsy.com/shop/Fractal9
Mat by Barefoot Yoga – barefootyoga.com

"You don't have to be great to start, but you have to start to be great."
– ZIG ZIGLAR

DOLPHIN POSE

Begin on your hands and knees. Align your wrists directly under your shoulders and your knees directly under your hips. Beginners can interlace their fingers.

Lower your elbows to the floor directly beneath your shoulders. Keep your forearms parallel to each other and to the side edges of your mat. Distribute your weight evenly across both forearms. Beginners will find interlacing their fingers helpful to prevent their elbows from splaying out.

Tuck your toes and lift your knees off the floor. Reach your pelvis up toward the ceiling, then draw your sit bones toward the wall behind you. Keep your knees bent as you lengthen your spine and broaden across your shoulder blades.

Then, gently begin to straighten your legs. Bring your torso and legs into the shape of an "A". Do not walk your feet closer to your hands—keep the extension of your whole body. If your upper back begins to round, bend your knees again until your spine is straight.

Draw your shoulder blades into your upper back ribs and toward your tailbone. Widen across your collarbones. Align your ears with your upper arms. Relax your head, but do not let it dangle. Gaze between your legs or toward your navel.

I find healthy eating especially difficult when out shopping. The mall is the worst for food choices. I always end up leaving there with a hankering for Cinnabon cinnamon rolls. Here is my solution. These protein bars are screaming with all the great flavors of a cinnamon roll, without all the guilt.

CINNAMON ROLL PROTEIN BARS

Makes 8 bars

1¼ cup Medjool dates, pitted
½ cup raisins
1 cup almonds
¼ cup walnuts
¼ cup cashews
½ teaspoon of vanilla
1 tablespoon cinnamon

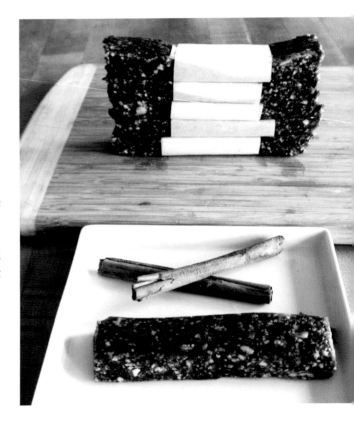

Add all ingredients to your food processor and pulse until fully incorporated.

Spread into a baking dish lined with parchment and chill for 1 hour before cutting. Store in an airtight container in the fridge or freezer.

"Belief consists in accepting the affirmations of the soul; unbelief, in denying them."
– RALPH WALDO EMERSON

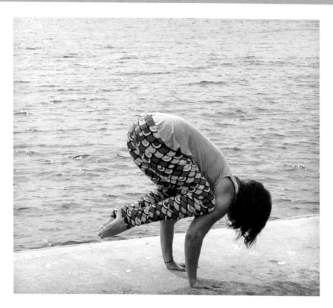

Top by Green Apple Activewear – greenappleactive.com
Leggings by Fractal9 – etsy.com/shop/Fractal9

CROW POSE

Start in Garland Pose (page 107) or low squat. Firm your hands down to the floor. Lift the hips high with your elbows at 90 degrees.

Place your knees as high up on your upper arms as you can, or squeeze the outer upper arms with your knees. Hug the knees and elbows in, exhale, and round strongly through the upper back, drawing your waist up using your abdominal muscles.

Then, squeezing in and up, bring the weight forward so the elbows end up straight over the wrist. Inhale, reach the heart forward, and let one foot come up (two if possible). Bring the heels and big toes together and lift the heels up over time towards the buttocks.

These brownies are so decadent you will not believe they are good for you.

HEALTHY DOUBLE-CHOCOLATE BROWNIES

Makes 8 brownies

1 cup whole raw almonds
1 cup whole raw walnuts
1 cup raw cacao powder
1½ cups Date Paste (page 164)

ICING
¾ cup raw cacao powder
¼ cup Date Paste (page 164)
½ cup full-fat coconut milk
¼ cup warm water
¼ cup coconut oil, melted

For the base

Place nuts in your food processor. Blend to a coarse meal. Add cacao powder and date paste. Blend to form brownie dough.

Press mixture evenly into a lined 8-inch square tray. It needs to be a few inches deep. Smooth out the top with a wet spatula. Place in the freezer while you make the icing.

For the icing

Add cacao powder, date paste, and coconut milk and blend to combine. Add in warm water and blend until smooth. Finally, add in melted coconut oil. Process until smooth and glossy.

Pour icing over the brownie base. Place in the fridge to firm up for 3 hours or overnight. Remove from the tray. Slice into desired number of brownies. Store in an airtight container in the fridge for up to 1 week or in the freezer for up to 1 month.

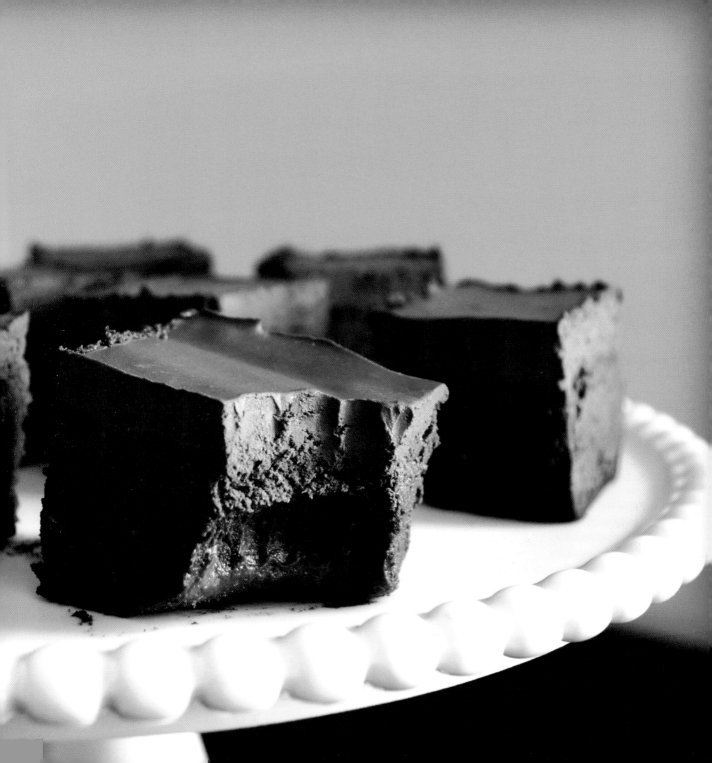

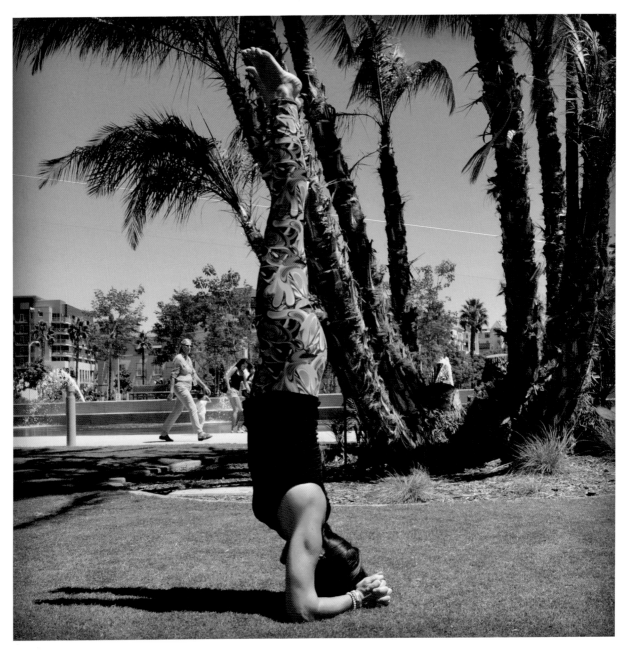

Tank by Be Present – bepresent.com
Leggings by Fractal9 – etsy.com/shop/Fractal9

> "Believe you can and you're halfway there."
> **– ATTRIBUTED TO THEODORE ROOSEVELT**

FOREARM BALANCE

Start off in Downward-Facing Dog (page 43). Your hands should be shoulder-width apart, You can either clasp your hands together, which is easier for beginners, or spread your fingers wide and grip the mat. Let your arm bones plug into their sockets, shoulder blades roll down the back, lower ribs corset in, navel pull in, core engage, and inner thighs rotate in.

Keeping the external rotation in your arms, slowly make your way onto your forearms. Forearms should be shoulder-width apart and parallel to each other. Let the head hang neutral. Push firmly into your hands and forearms and keep the elbows and upper arms squeezing in.

Walk your feet in as much as your flexibility allows. Look down and focus on the space in between your forearms. If you are having trouble keeping your elbows in, you can clasp your hands. This is easier for beginners; as you get comfortable with your shoulders, you can eventually flatten your palms.

Slowly lift one leg high into the air, bend the bottom leg, and lightly push off the foot. Keep the top leg energized and extended toward the sky while the bottom leg extends out. Both legs need to be active. Make sure not to let your face sink towards your mat. Push actively into your forearms and hands; keep the shoulders down and away from your ears. Try to keep the arms at 90 degrees.

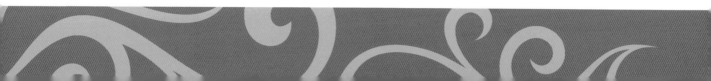

We all have bad days, bad weeks, moments of weakness. Having these on hand to grab during those times is a recipe for success. Who doesn't crave the classic chocolate chip cookie?

With 4 simple ingredients and 5 minutes you get these Healthy Chocolate Chip Cookies. Make these and you have a chewy chocolate chip cookie that is suitable for breakfast.

HEALTHY CHOCOLATE CHIP COOKIES

Makes 12 cookies

2 cups raw cashews
2 cups Medjool dates
1 teaspoon pure vanilla extract
3 tablespoon mini dark chocolate chips

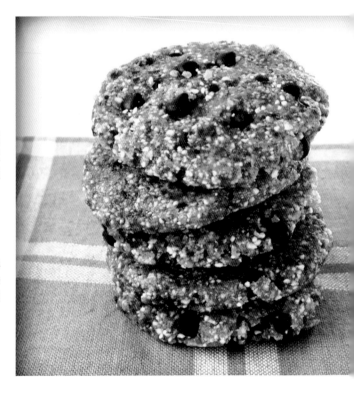

Add your cashews to a food processor and pulse until they resemble bread crumbs. Add your dates and vanilla. Make sure the pits have been removed and pulse until fully blended.

Stir in chocolate chips.

Roll approximately 2 tablespoons of the dough into a ball, then press flat. I do this on parchment paper. Place in an airtight container in the fridge or freezer until ready to serve.

SIDE CROW POSE

Begin in Mountain Pose (page 17). On your inhale, come into Chair Pose (page 67). With big toes and inner thighs touching, bend at the knees and lower the hips, keeping your tailbone down to eliminate the arching from the lower back. Shift the shins back to encourage the weight into the heels.

With hands together at the heart, twist to the right on the exhale breath, hooking the left elbow to the out-side of the right thigh, coming into side prayer twist (page 73) or Chair Pose twist.

Bring the knees in line with one another, press the right palm into the left, and roll the right shoulder back. Extend your heart away from your chest and lean the upper body back.

Staying in the twist, place both hands on the mat shoulder-distance apart, fingertips pointing away from the right thigh.

Bend the elbows to create a shelf. Bring the elbows directly on top of the wrists, lean forward, and begin to lift the shins up parallel to the mat, coming into Side Crow Pose. Keep the inner thighs squeezing in and the inner elbows firming in towards one another.

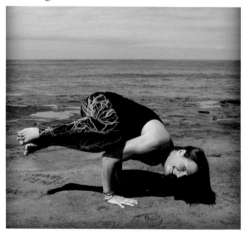

Top by Be Present – bepresent.com
Leggings by Fractal9 – etsy.com/shop/fractal9

"By believing passionately in something which still does not exist, we create it."
– NIKOS KAZANTZAKIS

Nothing lets me know it is autumn more than the smell of chai. The glorious aroma can draw us in and tempt us to fill our stomachs with seasonal treats. That is when this cookie saves the day.

It is a healthy cookie containing no added sugar, full of all things wholesome, ready in 5 minutes, and completely suitable for breakfast, snacks, lunch, dinner, and dessert.

HEALTHY VANILLA CHAI COOKIES

Makes 12 cookies

1 cup almonds
¼ cup walnuts
1 vanilla bean (pulp only)
2 teaspoons cinnamon
½ teaspoon ground ginger
½ teaspoon ground cardamom
¼ teaspoon ground allspice
⅛ teaspoon finely ground black pepper
1½ cups Medjool dates, pitted

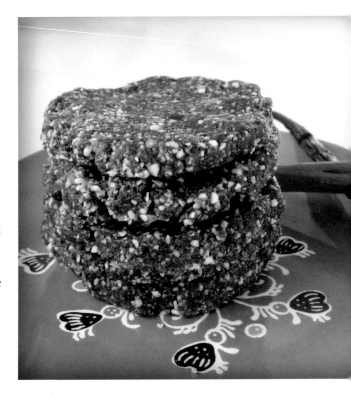

Add all ingredients to the food processor. Process until a thick dough forms.

Roll into balls and flatten on parchment paper. Store in the fridge or freezer in an airtight container.

FALLEN ANGEL

Begin in Mountain Pose (page 17). On your inhale, come into Chair Pose (page 67). With big toes and inner thighs touching, bend at the knees and lower the hips, keeping your tailbone down to eliminate the arching from the lower back. Shift the shins back to encourage the weight into the heels.

With hands together at the heart, twist to the right on the exhale breath, hooking the left elbow to the outside of the right thigh, coming into side prayer twist (page 73) or Chair Pose twist.

Bring the knees in line with one another, press the right palm into the left, and roll the right shoulder back. Extend your heart away from your chest and lean the upper body back.

Staying in the twist, place both hands on the mat shoulder-distance apart, fingertips pointing away from the right thigh.

Bend the elbows to create a shelf. Bring the elbows directly on top of the wrists, lean forward, and begin to lift the shins up parallel to the mat, coming into Side Crow Pose (page 205). Keep the inner thighs squeezing in and the inner elbows firming in towards one another.

From Side Crow Pose, turn gaze toward the bent knees and slowly lower the right temple onto the mat. Your right shoulder shouldn't touch the mat.

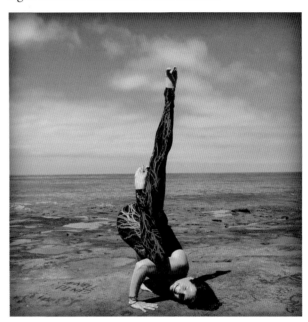

Top by Be Present – bepresent.com
Leggings by Fractal9 – etsy.com/shop/fractal9

"Change your thoughts and you change your world."
– NORMAN VINCENT PEALE

I don't know when it was decided peanut butter and jelly sandwiches were healthy, because they aren't. They are full of processed ingredients and sugar. These are made with 4 simple whole-food ingredients. Now you can have all the yummy comfort of peanut butter and jelly—in a healthy snack you can grab without any guilt.

HEALTHY PEANUT BUTTER AND JELLY COOKIES

Makes 12 cookies

2 cups peanuts
1 cup dates
⅛ cup water
1 tablespoon oat flour

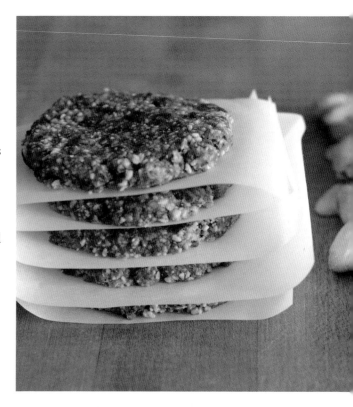

Place all ingredients in a food processor and process until a dough forms.

Roll into balls and press flat on parchment paper.

Serve! Store in an airtight container in the fridge and they last for weeks!

"Faith is not belief. Belief is passive. Faith is active."
– EDITH HAMILTON

PEACOCK POSE

Begin in Garland Pose (page 107). Place your hands on the floor between the knees with the palms down, fingertips pointing back towards the feet. Keep the hands touching together.

Bring your elbows together and place them on the abdomen. Try to keep the elbows close together throughout the pose.

Place your forehead on the mat in front of you. Straighten out both legs behind you. The body is now resting on the head, hands, and feet.

Lift your head and keep it up. Gradually shift the weight of your body forward, and as you do this, lift the feet. The body should be parallel to the floor. In the beginning, it is easier to lift each foot one at a time until you get the feeling for shifting the body weight forward and build up strength in the arms.

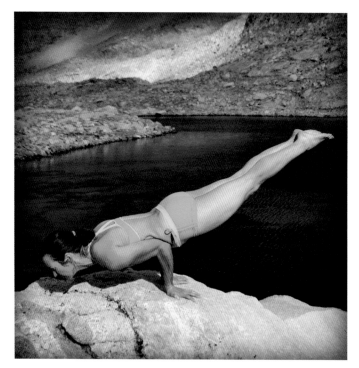

Outfit by Dragonfly – dragonfly-yogawear.com

Wow your friends with this refined sugar–free berry pie that is full of protein.

RAW BERRY TART

Makes 8 slices

CRUST:
2 cups Medjool dates, pitted
1 cup almond meal
1 cup unsweetened coconut flakes
¼ teaspoon sea salt
2 tablespoons water

FILLING:
2 cups fresh raspberries
2 cups cashews, soaked overnight and drained
2 tablespoons raw honey
¼ cup pure maple syrup
1 teaspoon vanilla extract
juice of 1 lime
¼ teaspoon sea salt
2 tablespoons coconut oil, melted

TOPPING:
½ cup raspberries, washed
½ cup strawberries, washed and sliced

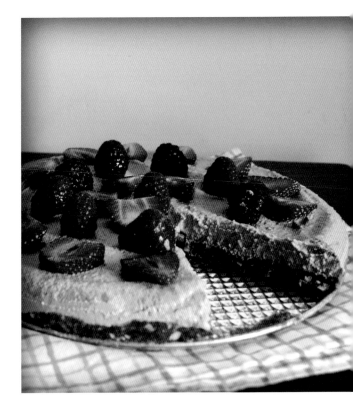

Place dates, almonds, coconut, and salt in a food processor and process at high speed. Add the water and pulse a couple of times. Test the crust by spooning a small amount in your hand and squeezing it. If it holds together nicely, it's ready. Scoop out crust mixture into a 10-inch springform pan and press firmly, making sure to press the crust up the sides of the pan as well. Evenly distribute the crust throughout the pan.

Place all filling ingredients except the coconut oil into your food processor. Blend at high speed until very smooth. This should take about a minute or two. Add the melted coconut oil and blend once more.

Pour the filling mixture out onto the crust and smooth with a spatula. Place in freezer until solid, about 1 hour.

Remove from freezer and arrange berries onto the tart. Serve immediately. Store leftovers in an airtight container in the fridge.

SUPPORTED HEADSTAND

Lace your fingers together and set the forearms on the floor, elbows at shoulder-width. Roll the upper arms slightly outward, but press the inner wrists firmly into the floor. Set the crown of your head on the floor. Press the bases of your palms together and snuggle the back of your head against the clasped hands.

Inhale and lift your knees off the floor. Carefully walk your feet closer to your elbows, heels elevated. Actively lift through the top thighs, forming an inverted "V". Firm the shoulder blades against your back and lift them toward the tailbone so the front torso stays as long as possible. This should help prevent the weight of the shoulders collapsing onto your neck and head.

Exhale and lift your feet away from the floor. As the legs (or thighs, if your knees are bent) rise perpendicular to the floor, firm the tailbone against the back of the pelvis. Turn the upper thighs in slightly and actively press the heels toward the ceiling, straightening the knees if you bent them to come up. The center of the arches should align over the center of the pelvis, which in turn should align over the crown of the head.

Once stable in this pose, you can try different leg variations as shown—just have fun and remember to breathe!

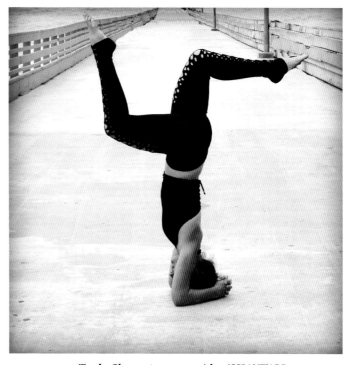

Top by Shantari – etsy.com/shop/SHANTARI
Leggings by 4TheWild – etsy.com/shop/4TheWild

"I always prefer to believe the best of everybody. It saves so much trouble."
– RUDYARD KIPLING

RAW VEGAN STRAWBERRY SHORTCAKE

Serves 4

1 cup Date Paste (page 164)
½ cup coconut flour
2 cups cashew meal
1 teaspoon vanilla
¼ cup water
Raw Vegan Whipped Cream (page 216)
fresh sliced strawberries

Place your date paste, coconut flour, cashew meal, vanilla, and water into a food processor and process until it resembles a dough.

Press dough into a medium baking dish prepared with parchment paper. Press the dough firmly into the bottom of the dish. Cover and place in the freezer for at least one hour to set.

Once set, remove from freezer and slice into serving-size pieces. Top with whipped cream and fresh sliced strawberries.

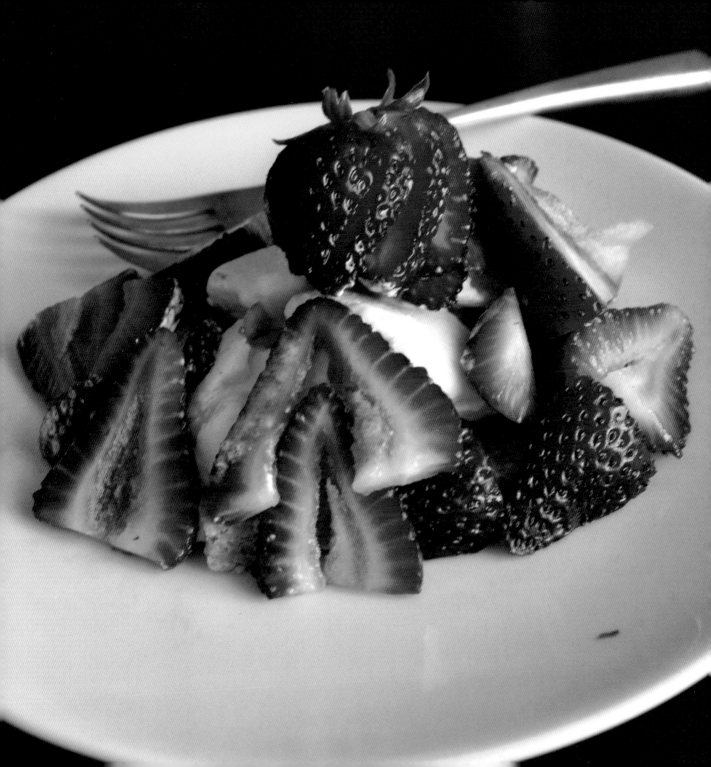

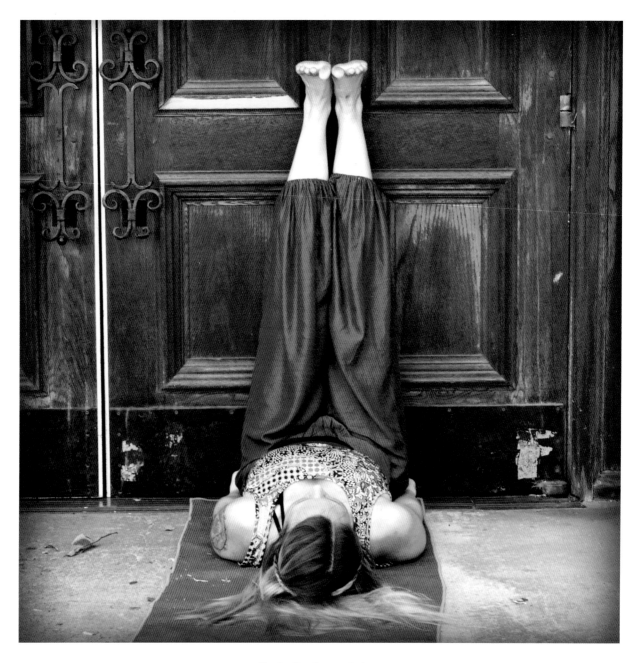

Top by Onzie – onzie.com
Pants By The High Thai – thehighthai.com

> "All our dreams can come true, if we have the courage to pursue them."
> **– WALT DISNEY**

LEGS-UP-THE-WALL POSE

Start seated with the left side of your body in contact with wall and your feet on the floor in front of you. Lie on your back and pivot so the backs of your legs press against the wall and the bottoms of your feet face up. Press your sit bones against or close to the wall and rest your back and head on the floor. Keep your body at a 90-degree angle.

Relax your head and neck in a neutral position and soften your face. Rest your hands on your belly or at your sides. Close your eyes and take slow, deep breaths through your nose for 5–15 minutes. To come out, push the bottoms of your feet into the wall, lifting your hips slightly. Slide your support out of the way if you used one. Gently roll to one side and stay for a few breaths before rising.

I use this in coffee, drinks, and desserts, or just as a dip for my fruit.

RAW VEGAN WHIPPED CREAM

Makes 1½ cups

1 (15-ounce) can of full-fat coconut milk
½ teaspoon stevia
1 teaspoon vanilla extract

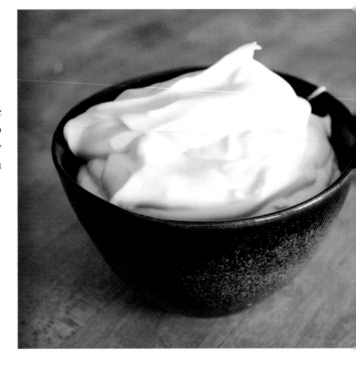

Place your can of coconut milk upside-down in the fridge overnight. Next day, turn the can right-side up and carefully open the can. Strain out all the watery liquid, leaving the solids. Mix your solids with stevia and vanilla. Whip up and serve.

TRIPOD HEADSTAND

Start close to a wall for support. Come on to your hands and knees into a Tabletop Pose (see page 111). Lower the crown of the head to the floor so that the head and the two hands form the points of a triangle.

Make sure your elbows are stacked on top of your wrists. Press your hands, including the finger and thumb pads, deeply into the earth. Breathe out and lift the pelvic floor and lower belly in and up. Keep the pelvic floor and belly engaged and your breath flowing into the chest and upper back.

Breathe out to lift the knees off the floor and begin to walk in. Try placing one knee onto your upper arm. Keep the spine long, the breath flowing, and the core engaged, then repeat with the other knee.

Begin to extend the legs up toward the ceiling. Keep hugging the legs into the midline and pressing out through the balls of the feet. Hug the legs in, with core deeply engaged and hands deeply connected to the earth, and then float the legs up.

> "A man's dreams are an index to his greatness."
> **– ZADOK RABINWITZ**

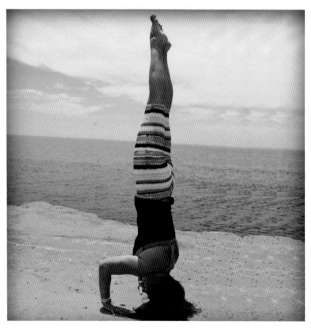

Tank Top by YOGASMOGA – yogasmoga.com
Leggings by Liza Jane Handmade – www.etsy.com/shop/lizajanehandmade
Jewelry by Indo Love Jewelry – www.etsy.com/shop/IndoLove

Making these cookies ahead of time ensures that you will have something wholesome on hand to turn to when you get a sweet tooth. All you need is 5 minutes. These are raw, vegan, gluten-free, and oh so good!

HEALTHY SNICKERDOODLE COOKIES

Makes 12 cookies

1 cup certified gluten-free rolled oats
1 cup almonds
1 vanilla bean (pulp only)
2 teaspoons cinnamon
12 Medjool dates
¼ cup water

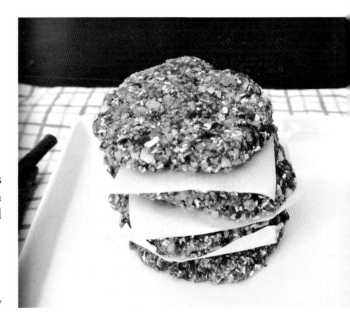

In the food processor, blend the oats and almonds until a bread-crumb consistency forms. Then, add in the rest of the ingredients to the food processor and pulse until a dough starts to form.

Roll into balls and then flatten them with your palm.

Store in an airtight container in the refrigerator. They store well in the freezer as well.

EPK

Start in Downward-Facing Dog (page 43), hands shoulder-width apart. Step your left foot far forward, past the outside of your left arm, and place it on the floor well in front of your left hand.

Bend your left elbow and twist your torso to the right, dropping the left shoulder and the whole left side of the torso as low as possible on your inner left thigh. Pressing your thigh toward your torso, slide your left upper arm and shoulder as far as you can underneath the back of the left thigh, just above the knee. Place the back of your thigh as high up as possible on the upper arm.

Keeping your weight centered between your hands. Start to creep your left foot forward along the floor, so more and more of the weight of the leg comes onto the arm; let the left foot naturally move a little to the left as you do this. When you can't walk the foot any farther forward without lifting it off the floor, straighten the knee as much as you can, powerfully reaching the foot forward and out to the left side.

Bending both elbows, shift your weight far forward between your hands until you can lift your back leg. Lift strongly until that leg is parallel to the floor; then, keeping the knee extended, press straight back through the ball of your foot.

Lift your chest until your torso is parallel to the floor, pressing strongly down through your inner hands to help maintain this position.

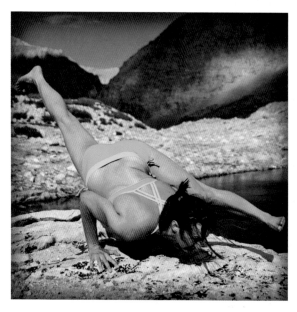

Outfit by dragonfly dragonfly-yogawear.com

> "Most great people have attained their greatest success just one step beyond their greatest failure."
> **– NAPOLEON HILL**

This is my favorite treat. Organic strawberries are so much sweeter than generic strawberries sold at supermarkets. I highly recommend them!

STRAWBERRY PARFAIT

Serves 2

1 cup Raw Vegan Whipped Cream (page 216)
2 cups fresh sliced strawberries
1 piece of 72% dark chocolate

Layer your parfait by alternating whipped cream and strawberries in a dessert bowl or glass. Top with chocolate piece and serve.

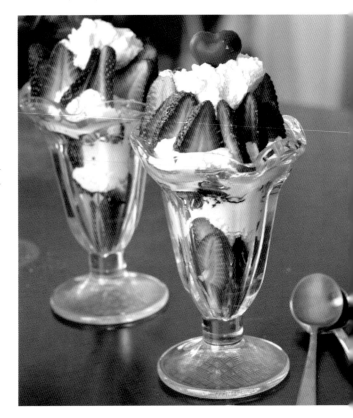

SEATED FORWARD FOLD

Begin in Mountain Pose (page 17) with your hands on your hips. Exhale as you bend forward at the hips, lengthening the front of your torso.

Bend your elbows and hold on to each elbow with the opposite hand. Let the crown of your head hang down. Press your heels into the floor as you lift your sit bones toward the ceiling. Turn the tops of your thighs slightly inward. Do not lock your knees.

If you can keep the front of your torso long and your knees straight, place your palms or fingertips on the floor beside your feet. Bring your fingertips in line with your toes and press your palms on the mat. Those with more flexibility can place their palms on the backs of their ankles or calves.

Engage your front thigh muscles and draw them up toward the ceiling. The more you engage your quadriceps, the more your rear thigh muscles will release.

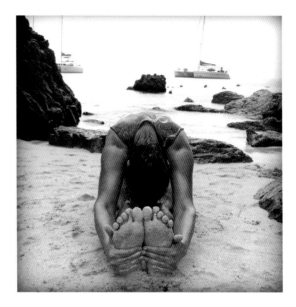

Outfit by Me and Harpua – etsy.com/shop/MeAndHarpua
Yoga Towel by EveryDay Yoga – etsy.com/shop/EverydayYoga

"As we are liberated from our own fear, our presence automatically liberates others."
– MARIANNE WILLIAMSON

You can still have your frozen treats while eating healthy. These shortcake pops are healthy enough for breakfast.

STRAWBERRY SHORTCAKE POPS

Serves 4

1½ cup puréed strawberries
¾ cup plain Greek yogurt
¾ cup unsweetened vanilla almond milk
¼ cup oat flour
3 tablespoons honey
½ cup cashew meal
⅓ cup Date Paste (page 164)

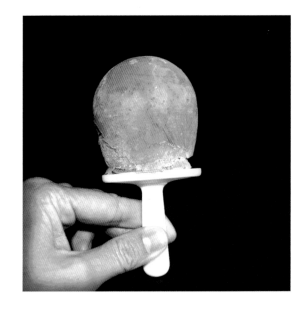

Wash your strawberries, slice the greens off, and place in a blender. Purée until smooth, then pour into a measuring cup. Measure 1 cup and place back inside the blender.

Add the yogurt, almond milk, oat flour, and honey into the blender and purée until smooth.

Mix together the cashew meal and the date paste. Make penny-sized pieces of mixture.

Place a few of the cookie pieces in the popsicle molds or ice cube tray. Pour strawberry mixture into popsicle molds (I use Zoku molds. For more information, visit zokuhome.com) or ice cube trays. Place more of the cookies in the molds. Freeze overnight.

"Do not look for approval except for the consciousness of doing your best."
– ANDREW CARNEGIE

CORPSE POSE

This is the final pose in yoga practice. Lie on your back and let your feet fall out to either side.

Bring the arms alongside the body, but slightly separated from the body, and turn the palms to face upwards.

Relax the whole body, including the face. Let the body feel heavy and the breath occur naturally.

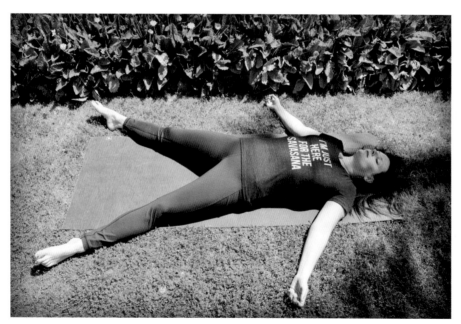

Shirt by: My Inner Fire – myinnerfire.com
Leggings by Vimmia – vimmia.com
Mat by Manduka – manduka.com

These bites of bliss are full of protein and nutrients—so much so that it is completely fine to eat one for breakfast!

VEGAN CARAMEL CHEESECAKE BITES

BASE:
1 cup almonds
1 cup pecans
4 tablespoons raw organic cacao powder
½ cup pitted Medjool dates
2 tablespoons coconut oil
1 teaspoon vanilla extract

FILLING:
2 cups raw cashews, soaked overnight in an
    airtight container
1 cup organic zucchini, peeled and diced
1 teaspoon stevia or 2 tablespoons raw honey
4 tablespoons coconut oil
½ cup maple syrup
1 teaspoon vanilla extract
¼ teaspoon sea salt

Caramel Sauce (page 162)

Put all the ingredients for the base crust in a food processor and process until it has a wet and crumbly texture. Divide evenly into a lined 12-cavity muffin pan and press down firmly. Put the cheesecake pan in the freezer to harden the crust while you prepare the cheesecake filling.

Put all the ingredients for the filling into a blender and blend until smooth and creamy. You want to run several cycles and scrape down the blender because you want it as creamy as you can get, so plan on several minutes here.

Remove the cheesecake pan from the freezer and evenly distribute the filling on top of each crust. Place back in the freezer to set for 1 hour.

Top with caramel sauce and serve. Store in an airtight container in the fridge for up to 1 week. They can also be frozen for up to 30 days for future serving.

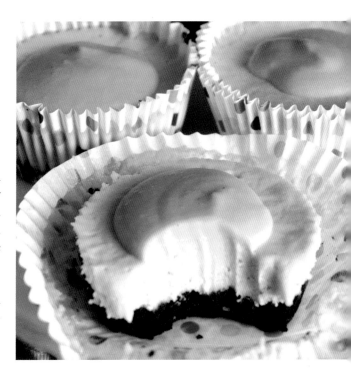

> "Happiness comes of the capacity to feel deeply, to enjoy simply, to think freely, to risk life, to be needed."
> **– STORM JAMESON**

PARTNER YOGA

Yoga is a lot of fun with friends. Partner yoga is an amazing way to deepen your practice. Two people rely on each other to keep balanced, aligned, and focused in a pose.

When done correctly, partner yoga elevates each person's individual yoga practice, and also strengthens relationships between its participants. It's a great thing to do with your significant other, but also with a friend or family member. The image to the right is of me and my daughter.

In partner yoga, participants benefit from a bigger sense of self-awareness. When you practice alone, you may be completely unaware of what your front ribs are doing, but the moment someone puts their hands on you, your consciousness is drawn to that part of your body. Your practice begins to deepen a lot faster.

I would encourage you to grab a friend and practice together. There are limitless resources online to guide you through poses.

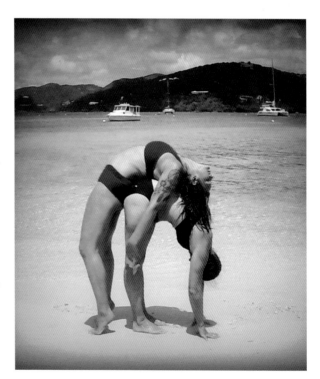

Suits by Dragonfly – dragonfly-yogawear.com

COOKING MEASUREMENT EQUIVALENTS

Cups	Tablespoons	Fluid Ounces
⅛ cup	2 Tbsp.	1 fl. oz.
¼ cup	4 Tbsp.	2 fl. oz.
⅓ cup	5 Tbsp. + 1 tsp.	
½ cup	8 Tbsp.	4 fl. oz.
⅔ cup	10 Tbsp. + 2 tsp.	
¾ cup	12 Tbsp.	6 fl. oz.
1 cup	16 Tbsp.	8 fl. oz.

Cups	Fluid Ounces	Pints/Quarts/Gallons
1 cup	8 fl. oz.	½ pint
2 cups	16 fl. oz.	1 pint = ½ quart
3 cups	24 fl. oz.	1½ pints
4 cups	32 fl. oz.	2 pints = 1 quart
8 cups	64 fl. oz.	2 quarts = ½ gallon
16 cups	128 fl. oz.	4 quarts = 1 gallon

Other Helpful Equivalents

1 Tbsp.	3 tsp.
8 oz.	½ lb.
16 oz.	1 lb.

METRIC MEASUREMENT EQUIVALENTS

Approximate Weight Equivalents

Ounces	Pounds	Grams
4 oz.	¼ lb.	113 g
5 oz.		142 g
6 oz.		170 g
8 oz.	½ lb.	227 g
9 oz.		255 g
12 oz.	¾ lb.	340 g
16 oz.	1 lb.	454 g

Approximate Volume Equivalents

Cups	US Fluid Ounces	Milliliters
⅛ cup	1 fl. oz.	30 ml
¼ cup	2 fl. oz.	59 ml
½ cup	4 fl. oz.	118 ml
¾ cup	6 fl. oz.	177 ml
1 cup	8 fl. oz.	237 ml

Other Helpful Equivalents

½ tsp.	2½ ml	
1 tsp.	5 ml	
1 Tbsp.	15 ml	

INDEX

ABOUT THE AUTHOR

Christi Silbaugh is the author of *Gluten-Free Made Easy* and of *Gourmet Cooking for Two*. She also writes for numerous media outlets like *Activewear USA Magazine, Glam Media,* and *Federated Media.* Sharing recipes, yoga tips, and her personal journey, her popular blog *"Mom, What's for Dinner?"* has over 2.5 million readers. For couples, her playful romance food blog *"Gourmet Cooking for Two"* offers spicy tips for the kitchen.

After surviving cancer, her love of food married her passion for being healthy. Since receiving her 200-Hour Yoga One Teacher Certification in 2014, Christi is committed to helping heal the world through conscious healthy eating and moving the body. She also has started a nonprofit called We Are Warriors, which brings free recovery yoga to past and present cancer patients.

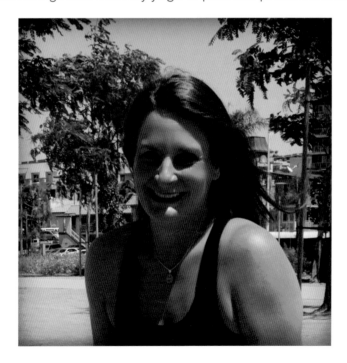

0 26575 15525 9